VITAMIN D
PRESCRIPTION

The Healing Power of the Sun & How It Can Save Your Life

Eric Madrid MD

ISBN: 1-4392-2946-5
ISBN-13: 9781439229460

Visit www.booksurge.com to order additional copies.

CONTENTS

DEDICATION

I dedicate this book to my patients who have inspired me to search for ways to help keep them healthy and disease free. Also, I dedicate it to my grandfather, James B. Shaffer (1918-2007) who encouraged me to seek for truth in all I do.

SPECIAL THANKS

Special thanks to my lovely wife, Whanda, who encouraged me and never complained about all the nights and weekends I spent on this book. For our two boys, Joshua and Jonathan, this is the key to health and longevity; learn it well.

Special thanks to the Vitamin D Council (http://www.vitamindcouncil. org/)—a group of scientists whose hard work and dedication have helped spread the word about the health benefits of vitamin D. These scientists and their research will save more lives than any other health movement or pharmaceutical medicine ever has, second only, perhaps, to penicillin. Specifically, I would like to thank Cedric Garland, DrPH, and Frank Garland, PhD, of the University of California, San Diego, whose studies have inspired me to learn all I could on the subject, and Michael Holick MD, PhD, of Boston University Medical Center, whose research is amazing. When the Nobel Prize is given out for vitamin D research, Dr. Michael Holick will surely be first in line. I am simply a messenger who is helping to spread the lifesaving information to the masses. Also, a special thanks for Carole Baggerly of Grass Roots Health who is also spreading the word (www.grassrootshealth. org) about vitamin D.

Also, I would like to thank my editor, Cindy Fleming-Wood. Your suggestions and feedback are much appreciated. Thanks to Jennifer M. Clare (clare_jenniferm@yahoo.com) who illustrated various images in this book.

SECTION I:
INTRODUCTION

"If I have seen further, it is by standing on the shoulders of giants."
- Sir Isaac Newton 1642–1727

I remember going to the beautiful beaches of Southern California as a young child. I was a California native; little did I know that growing up where the sun shines 330 days or more a year was the exception and not the rule. I assumed everyone had access to a beach, perfect weather, and Disneyland. Having a suntan was simply the result of living in Southern California and was not something one had to work for, especially a child. Certainly, Southern Californians were not deficient in vitamin D, the sunshine vitamin, or were they?

I was born in 1972 to teenage parents. Times were tumultuous, to say the least. The Vietnam War, a conflict that killed 58,169 Americans (11,465 were teenagers) and over one million Vietnamese, was tearing the country apart. Fortunately for me, my dad avoided the draft.

The oil crisis started when I was about 1 ½ years old and resulted from OPEC's decision to not to ship oil to any country that supported Israel in the Yom Kippur war. Gasoline prices went from 35 cents a gallon to a high of almost 60 cents per gallon. Up until that point, Americans had enjoyed the luxury of cheap gasoline and fast cars. Now, Americans lined up just so they could fill up their gas tanks. Topping off gas tanks was discouraged due to the shortage, so there was a $5 minimum purchase.

The political landscape was in an upheaval. Distrust of government was at an all-time high. Richard Nixon, the least popular president to date, was in office and was soon to be impeached for lying about his role in the Watergate scandal.

On December 23, 1971, while in the midst of the Vietnam War, President Nixon started another war of which few were aware. Even today, few know about it. He sought no approval from Congress before starting this war, a battle that would take place on U.S. soil. He called for a War against *Cancer*. However, almost 40 years later, 1 in 3 women and 1 in 2 men in America are still diagnosed with cancer at some point in their lifetimes.

> ## "Seven million people worldwide will die from cancer, including 506,650 Americans"

In 2008, approximately 506,650 people died from cancer in the USA. Worldwide, nearly 7 million people died, according to the World Health Organization. According to the American Cancer Society, 170,000 of the annual cancer deaths in the U.S. could be prevented if people quit smoking. Worldwide, around 2.5 million lives could be saved. The war against cancer is a war we have been losing—until now.

What if this trend could be reversed? What if colon cancer, breast cancer, ovarian cancer, and prostate cancer rates could be reduced by 20% to 60%, or more—even in the absence of smoking cessation? Would we consider the war on cancer a success? How would your life change?

What if you could prevent cancer from affecting you in the future? What if you could prevent your spouse, friends, siblings, or even your children from developing cancer? Cancer is one of the scariest words a person can ever hear. Just about everyone knows someone who has been affected by cancer. Would reading the rest of this book be worth their lives? Would it be worth your life?

By the 1970s, the measles vaccine had become a common immunization for young children. While the incidence of measles was decreasing, the number of children who developed measles plummeted after routine vaccination became available. At the time, the connection between infection and cancer was beginning to be studied and it was soon realized that some cancers could be induced by viruses.

In 2006, Merck marketed the Gardasil® vaccine. Gardasil is the first "anticancer" vaccine, designed to protect young women from the human papillomavirus, or HPV, a wart virus present in women with cervical cancer. More will be discussed regarding this issue in the cervical cancer section. However, studies show that vitamin D may help prevent cervical cancer—with no side effects.

If physicians, with the support of health insurance companies, recommended that all their patients be screened for vitamin D deficiency, enormous public health benefits would be realized. Doctors could advise those who were deficient to take vitamin D supplements. Tens of thousands of lives could be saved annually. Also, billions of healthcare dollars could possibly be saved each year in cancer treatments. This simple strategy could improve success in our war against cancer.

In 1928, Alexander Fleming serendipitously discovered the antibiotic, penicillin. This discovery occurred after mold contaminated his science experiments. Twelve years later, English scientists isolated the active ingredient of penicillin and found that doctors could use it to treat World War II soldiers with infections. Shortly thereafter, death rates from infections diminished tremendously. People no longer died from blood infections, urine infections, and pneumonia as they once had. There is now research to suggest that the influenza virus, pneumonia and even tuberculosis, can be prevented or treated more efficiently with vitamin D supplementation. You will read more about this later in the book.

Computed tomography (CT) and the magnetic resonance imaging (MRI) machines were invented and made available for public use in the 1970s. For the first time, doctors had the ability to take images of the inside of human bodies, which simplified diagnostics and made visualization of cancers more certain.

The "art of medicine" began to lose its competitive edge while the "science of medicine" took front row. However, 40 years later, there is concern that cumulative radiation from CT exams may actually cause some cancers and that by 2030, 2% of all cancers may have been induced by CT imaging exams. Fortunately ultrasounds and MRIs are radiation-free, so it is likely that these will become more widely used over time.

In the 1970s, doctors started to realize the link between high blood pressure, heart disease, and stroke. Few would have thought that a vitamin D deficiency might be related to those illnesses. In addition, doctors then realized that treating high blood pressure could decrease one's chance of having a heart attack. Forty years later, vitamin D appears to do both—lower blood pressure and prevent heart attacks. This will be discussed more in Section V.

It was also time for a pill to be commonly prescribed for diabetes treatment; until then, the only available option was an insulin shot. Studies show that diabetics are more likely to be vitamin D deficient when compared to

3

nondiabetics. Vitamin D actually helps make your insulin more effective.

Those with thinning bones (osteopenia) and osteoporosis also have lower vitamin D levels than those with stronger bones. Lack of vitamin D weakens the bones and can increase risks of falls and injuries. Other studies have shown that people who suffer from chronic pain, nonspecific muscle aches, and fibromyalgia also tend to have lower serum vitamin D levels than those who don't.

Rickets, a disease caused by vitamin D deficiency was rampant until the 1930s. Rickets causes weak bones and malformation of bones in infants and children. Fortunately, in the 1930s, it was discovered that a daily dose of cod liver oil—or simply increased sunlight exposure—could prevent the dreaded disease. Ironically, it would take almost 80 years for doctors and scientists to realize that rickets was only the tip of the iceberg when it came to the myriad of diseases that vitamin D could prevent (Figure 1).

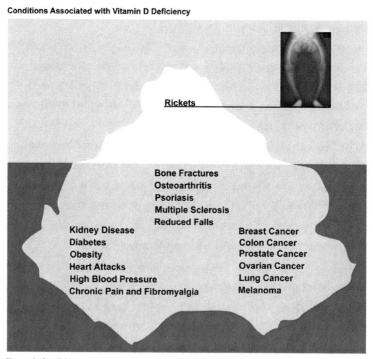

Figure 1. Conditions associated with vitamin D deficiency. Illustrated by Jennifer M. Clare.

In the 1980s, scientists discovered an inverse relationship between sun exposure and cancer incidence. Simply stated, those with more sunshine exposure had fewer cancers, excluding nonmelanoma skin cancer. The significance of this was yet to be determined. You will read more about this later.

Would good old-fashioned medicine be lost with our technological advancements? Would the health benefits of a noon walk in the sun be buried in the memory hole of past generations? Would the health benefits of cod liver oil be forgotten?

To return to my childhood stories—I spent a lot of time at the beach until my teenage years. When I was 7 years old, I remember driving down the San Gabriel (605) freeway with my mom on our way from Whittier to Long Beach, both suburbs of Los Angeles.

Upon arrival at the beaches of the Pacific Coast, my mother, who is of French-German heritage, would slop on the Coppertone suntan oil from head to toe. She would then lie out on the beach and roast like a chicken on a George Foreman rotisserie grill, rolling over every 45 minutes or so to ensure an even tan. Brown skin was her goal (as well as that of thousands of others), and with enough patience and perseverance, many achieved it with Coppertone.

As I look at the Coppertone ad (Figure 2) now, 30 years later, it amazes me that they used to actually have magazine advertisements and billboards of this girl plastered on the sides of the freeways of Southern California, Florida, and I am sure numerous other locations where sunbathing was common. Today, this ad, which exposed a child's buttocks, would be criminal. In either case, she was unknowingly promoting the generation of vitamin D and cancer prevention.

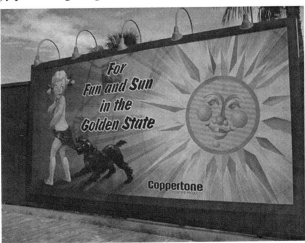

Figure 2. Updated Coppertone advertisement, as seen at Disney's Adventure Park, California.

I would play in the waves, dig holes in the sand, make sandcastles, and catch the ever-elusive sand crabs. I would make friends instantly and could easily spend 8 hours in the sun. Being also of Hispanic heritage, I was fortunate to tan very nicely; I rarely got a sunburn. My skin would turn golden brown, without the use of any suntan lotion.

Of course, what fun was a trip to the beach without mischievousness? I would stroll along the shore in search of the slimiest, grossest, brown or green seaweed in hopes of scaring my mom. I would bring the underwater plant life to where she lay, and drop it on her as she rested with her eyes shut. I usually ended up getting yelled at and would simply go back to splashing in the waves. The whole time, my brown skin was making vitamin D, which would circulate in my blood to the organs of my body and ultimately help me build strong bones and prevent disease.

I had great times at the beach! There was no culture of fear back then. I am sure there were kidnappings, but they rarely made it onto the evening news and people were not afraid of one another. If anything, they looked out for each other. In addition, fear of skin cancer was not as prevalent. Perhaps it is the fear we now have that keeps our children indoors more and has led to the vitamin D deficiency epidemic.

Little did I know, my mom was also optimizing her levels of Vitamin D, which would ultimately have numerous health benefits that would protect her from numerous diseases in the future—the diseases we didn't know much about back in the 1970s. When I compare my mom's health to my grandmother's health at the same age, my mom has definitely had fewer medical problems than my sun-sensitive, fair-skinned grandmother who avoided sunlight exposure.

From the shore, I saw the surfboarders and the boogie boarders, wondering if I would ever be able to do that. Although I figured out boogie boarding, I have not yet surfed. However, as with many other life goals, it is just a matter of time. Unfortunately, those *JAWS* movies have entered into my psyche so I need to do a little "brain reprogramming" before I put on a wet suit, lay on a surfboard, and look like a seal from below the surface of the water—a shark's eye view of the world.

Few realized back then that surfers, sunbathers, and lifeguards were actually practicing preventive medicine. Their blood levels of vitamin D were at optimal levels, ranging from 50 ng/ml (125 nmol/L) to 80 ng/ml (200 nmol/L).

It would be 30 years before we realized the benefits of sunlight. Although nonmelanoma skin cancers would likely become more prevalent among the sun worshipers, their rates of breast cancer, colon cancer, and prostate cancers, among others, would be less common. In addition, they would have fewer metabolic bone diseases.

Many years passed, I had forgotten about my childhood days at the beach. I did not realize the significance they would have later on in my life.

In 1994, I started my studies at UCLA. I was excited to attend a university that had worldwide recognition and enjoyed an excellent reputation in the sciences and medicine. I was on schedule to become a physician and wanted to make sure my future was on track. I decided to major in microbiology and molecular genetics. Genetics was an emerging field in the health sciences. The human genome project was underway and the whole human existence and decoding of human deoxyribonucleic acid (DNA) was imminent. Once this was complete, we hoped to finally understand cancers and other diseases and take measures to reverse these horrible conditions. Perhaps the cure for cancer lay in decoding the human genome.

I had a wonderful experience at UCLA. The university was huge and the sun shone 330 days a year. The diversity of the students on campus made it more enjoyable. Students got great exercise simply walking from one class to the other. It took several hours just to walk around the campus perimeter.

Studying microbiology and genetics was quite thorough and inclusive; we learned nearly everything about how genes are controlled and regulated. One year of biochemistry classes taught me biology at the molecular level; specifically, how one molecule interacts with another molecule. However, I did not learn anything about vitamin D and its influence on cell regulation. Scientists were just discovering this information, and it was not in the textbooks at the time. Researchers knew little about vitamin D and its ability to regulate cell growth and division. However, my education on genetics and how genes are controlled formed a strong foundation that would prepare me for my future research on vitamin D.

After graduating from UCLA, I attended The Ohio State University School of Medicine. While a student, I married my beautiful wife, Whanda, and we had two sons, Joshua and Jonathan. As intense as my studies were at The Ohio State, the only mention of vitamin D was the fact that, if it is too low, a person can develop rickets. There was no talk about sunlight, vitamin D, and cancer prevention. I did learn that vitamin D was needed for adequate calcium to be properly absorbed; however, no specific blood level was suggested. As I look back, I realize that my young family and I most definitely spent our years in Ohio being vitamin D deficient.

While my wife and I took multivitamins, the dose of vitamin D in most multivitamins, including Centrum and Centrum Silver, are severely inadequate to prevent anything but rickets in the majority who take them.

I graduated from medical school in 2002. Columbus was a beautiful city and we enjoyed the changes of the seasons. The huge maple tree leaves turned color each fall to a brilliant reddish-orange color. Seeing this was a nice experience, one rarely appreciated while living in Southern California.

Columbus, Ohio, was a great place to raise a family. The community where we lived was safe and very family-oriented. Crimes were minimal and the landscape of Columbus and the surrounding communities was majestic. We had a nice condo close to the university.

It was difficult not having family nearby and raising young ones. Fortunately, we "adopted" a grandmother in Columbus who would watch the boys so my wife and I could go out together on an occasional date. It was difficult not having the children see their grandparents on a regular basis. After graduation from medical school, the Madrid family would finally head back to the land of sunshine, blue skies, and beaches. We were happy to return to California where our families were. Surely now our blood vitamin D levels would rise and I would start my family medicine residency.

Residency is what a medical student does after graduation. Most residencies take 3 to 5 years. This provides newly graduated physicians with additional training in the specialty of their choice. It is one of the steps required for a physician to become a board certified physician in his or her specialty. Family medicine, pediatrics, and internal medicine specialties require 3 years of specialized training after graduating from medical school.

It is a shame that recent years have seen a significant decline in the number of medical students entering into primary care. One reason is the rising costs of medical education. Most medical students are now graduating medical school with a student debt of over $150,000. In addition, rising malpractice costs can be as much as $12,000 per year. As a result, most medical students are choosing to enter specialties and subspecialties (neurosurgery, orthopedics, cardiology, etc.) where they can command twice the income of primary care physicians. I have a lot of respect for those medical school graduates who enter family medicine, internal medicine, and pediatrics in spite of the lower income.

"Disease prevention and health maintenance are what really matter"

Disease prevention and health maintenance are what really matter. It is important that people have access to primary care physicians who can help prevent heart disease, diabetes, diabetic complications, kidney disease, and strokes, which if acquired, require the care of specialists. This is where primary care medicine and disease prevention take center stage.

A first-year resident is called an intern. Residents do rotations in cardiology, nephrology (kidney specialists), orthopedics, hospital medicine, women's health, ob-gyn, surgery, and other areas, including dermatology. These rotations help a young physician learn the specifics of each specialty. After my year of internship, a 2004 law prohibited residents from working more than 80 hours per week. Prior to that, there were weeks when I spent almost 100 hours working at the hospital.

During my second year of residency, I did a 4-week rotation at a dermatologist's office. Dr. Piel (name changed) was was a fabulous physician. I learned a lot about skin cancers, rashes, and psoriasis during my 4 weeks at Dr. Piel's office; this training would become my foundation. Curiously, Dr. Piel would walk into the office every day with white sunscreen smudged all over his face. He would go through the day and would not really rub it in very thoroughly. He would walk in and out of patient rooms examining their rashes, skin moles, or infections with sunscreen all over his face. New patients would look at him strangely; old patients were happy to see him, as they were used to it.

One day, I finally got the nerve to ask him why he did not rub the sunscreen in. He responded, "I am trying to protect my skin—everyone should wear this much sunscreen on their face and arms to prevent skin cancer."

9

The message to his patients was also clear; he led by example. I am certain that if we had checked Dr. Piel's blood level for vitamin D, we would have found he was severely deficient. Did he have any idea that he was vitamin D deficient? Did he take vitamin D supplements? I don't know—but my intuition tells me probably not. If he was aware of the vitamin D deficiency epidemic, he did not share that knowledge with me.

> ## "All this sunscreen use may actually be promoting more deadly cancers while preventing fewer deadly skin cancers"

In my opinion, this type of sunscreen use is contributing to vitamin D deficiency epidemics. While protecting skin against sunburns is important, slopping on a ton of sunscreen may be dangerous to one's health. All this sunscreen use may actually be promoting more deadly cancers while preventing fewer deadly skin cancers. Studies have shown that some sunscreens actually increase the risk of developing melanoma. We will explore this more in the melanoma section. Extensive sunscreen use is only part of the problem though.

Overall, children and adults are spending less and less time outdoors— we do less biking, walking, gardening, and playing ball. Today, Europeans and Americans spend more time indoors on the computer, playing video games, or watching television. As a result, we are absorbing less ultraviolet light (UV-B) through our skin. We can now run 3 miles (~5km) and bike 15 miles (~45 km) without ever leaving our homes or apartments.

While exercise is beneficial to our heart and lungs, we are completely eliminating the benefits that sunshine has to offer us when we do those activities indoors. Few families take bike rides or walks together anymore. This has become an activity of the past. I heard a story of a physician who spent his lunchtime taking a noon walk near his office. Because people recognized him, cars would pull over frequently and ask him if he needed a ride. The physician commented that walking had become so rare, that when others saw him, they assumed his car had broken down or that something was wrong. In 2005, I went into private practice. I started to learn about vitamin D deficiency and the associated problems. I eventually spent years researching the benefits of sunlight exposure, vitamin D testing, supplementation, disease prevention, and worked to spread the word. I read and reviewed hundreds of scientific journal articles, newspaper reports, and textbooks so I could put together a complete health guide for patients.

The way I see it, people need to take personal responsibility for their health. As mentioned, the number of primary care physicians is decreasing while the number of specialists is increasing. We have a disease care system that rewards physicians with more money to treat patients with disease and illness. Physicians who want to practice preventive medicine, help reverse heart disease, and prevent diabetes in patients through dietary changes and exercise are paid less. Preventing disease with safe and adequate sunshine exposure and vitamin D supplementation is an important step in the right direction. Vitamin D is a supplement that scientists and physicians are now realizing can improve our health in significant way. A paradigm shift has begun!

The culmination of my research is the publication this book. This is the first edition and my hopes are that it lays the foundation for you and your family in your search for optimal health and longevity.

SECTION II:
RICKETS, VITAMIN D DEFICIENCY, AND GENES

"It is much more important to know what sort of a patient has a disease than what sort of disease a patient has."
- Sir William Osler (1849–1919)

Few adults today recognize the term *rickets*. Some can at least identify that it has something to do with the bones. Ask your parents or grandparents, and they can likely tell you a story about being forced to swallow a teaspoon or two of cod liver oil as a child. They will usually make sour-looking faces as they describe the experience. They may not have known why they were taking it, simply that their parents made them and that it was "good for your bones." They will also tell you it tasted horrible. Scientists in the 1930s discovered that supplementing the diet with cod liver provided enough vitamin D to prevent rickets, the dreaded bone disease of the day.

Like other future physicians, I learned in medical school that rickets was a disease caused by vitamin D deficiency. Furthermore, I learned that today in developed countries, such as the U.S. and countries in Europe, few people suffer from rickets, a "disease of antiquity." Vitamin deficiency was not something that we saw anymore; it had been conquered as a "disease of the past."

If I had asked my professors or chief resident at the time to measure a vitamin D level in a patient, they would have thought I was crazy. Surely, no one was deficient in vitamin D in the United States. Not even in Ohio. Even if they were, a simple multivitamin or a glass of milk would have been sufficient to correct it. Little did I know at the time that vitamin D deficiency was a silent epidemic among many people and that a severe deficiency, which causes rickets, was making a comeback in the U.S. The childhood disease results in malformation and weakening of the bones. According to Mayo-Clinic.com, rickets has the following signs:

- **Skeletal deformities**—Bowed legs, abnormal curvature of the spine, pelvic deformities, and breastbone projection in the chest
- **Fragile bones**—Those with rickets are prone to fractures
- **Impaired growth**—Shorter stature and limbs
- **Dental problems**—Defective teeth, increased cavities, poor enamel and delayed formation of teeth
- **Bone pain**—Dull, aching pain or tenderness in the spine, pelvis, and legs
- **Muscle weakness**—Muscle pain and increased fall risk

Since calcium and phosphorus absorption in the intestines require vitamin D, a lack of calcium absorption ultimately results in poor bone mineralization and weak bones.

In recent years, several other variations of rickets have been discovered, some of which are *not* due to vitamin D deficiency. A second cause of rickets is due to undernourishment, which results in diminished calcium and other mineral intake. In this scenario, the person has plenty of vitamin D synthesis from sunlight exposure, but is unable to absorb the calcium due to a deficient diet. We usually see this type of rickets in places like Africa, Haiti, and South and Central America where sunlight exposure is adequate but mineral intake is limited, especially calcium intake.

In 2007 and 2008, I had the privilege of visiting the beautiful Caribbean island of Haiti with fellow physicians on a medical mission trip with the Haiti Endowment Fund. We provided medical care to children and adults in the countryside villages. I witnessed firsthand a community where basic nutrition was lacking. We visited a community marketplace that sold mud pies. Mud pies are literally rocks that people ate so they could get adequate iron and other minerals. Pregnant women especially would eat these in order to provide nutrients for their unborn babies. While I am not certain they contained calcium, this illustrates the extremes people will go to in order to get basic minerals for their health.

A third type of rickets results from a genetic defect that results in defective production of vitamin D metabolites. Others may have Type I hereditary vitamin D-dependent rickets or Type II hereditary vitamin D-dependent rickets, which only respond to certain forms of vitamin D. The person has plenty of vitamin D in his/her blood and adequate calcium in the diet, but the cells of the body are unable to recognize the vitamin D. The result is the same as having a vitamin D deficiency, and abnormal bone formation results.

Rickets is rare in the United States and other industrialized countries. However in recent years, the number of cases has increased. Before and during the early 1900s, rickets was common in those who lived in poverty or lived in the northern latitudes where the sun does not shine much. During the days of the industrial revolution, when people burned coal for fuel, the skies were more polluted. The ultraviolet waves (UV-B) did not reach the skin so vitamin D synthesis was inadequate. This has led some vitamin D experts to suggest that Charles Dickens perhaps described a child with rickets in his depiction of Tiny Tim, when he wrote, "Alas for Tiny Tim... he bore a little crutch, and had his limbs supported by an iron frame!" He wrote his book in 1899, when rickets was present in about 80% of children in some cities.

There were many theories and ideas as to why rickets developed. Physicians of the day were not entirely certain, but suspected that hygiene and sunlight had something to do with it (Figure 3).

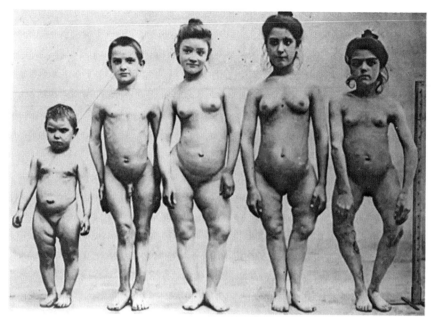

Figure 3. Children from Paris with rickets. (National Institute of Health,
http://www.nlm.nih.gov/exhibition/cesarean/images/rickets.jpg).

Descriptions of rickets appear in old medical scrolls and textbooks that go back over 2,000 years. Although people did not understand the cause at the time, the effects on human development were clear. Below is a list of physicians of antiquity who recognized the condition.

Soranus of Ephesus (98 AD-138 AD), a Greek "family doctor" who practiced gynecology, obstetrics, and pediatrics, lived in the second century AD. He practiced medicine in Rome during the rule of Trajan (98-117 AD) and Hadrian (117–138 AD). He described a bone condition in Roman children of the day, which was later determined to be a description of rickets. He blamed Roman mothers for poor nourishment and poor hygiene of their children as the cause of their bony malformations. He was not successful in treating it.

Claudius Galen (131 AD–201 AD) made many contributions to medicine; a vein in the brain bears his name. He was the first to identify human veins and arteries and their different functions. In addition, he performed cataract surgeries almost 1,900 years before surgeons tried again.

He was the court physician to the great Roman emperor, Marcus Aurelius. Galen wrote many articles on medicine and helped set the standard for modern medicine. He described Roman children's bony malformations, which were later determined to be rickets.

Daniel Whistler (1618–1684), an English physician, in 1645 published the first description of rickets in his doctoral thesis at the University of Leyden.

Francis Glisson (1597–1677), a British physician and anatomy expert, helped define liver anatomy. He published *A Treatise of the Rickets— Being a Diseas(e) common to Children,* which better characterized rickets.

Armand Trousseau of France (1801–1867), a French internist, stated in 1861 that rickets was caused by lack of sunlight, a faulty diet, and that cod liver oil could treat it. However, this information was unrealized for almost 70 years. Unfortunately, he developed stomach cancer and died.

Edward Mellanby (1884–1955), an English physician, showed in 1919 that cod liver oil, when given to dogs, could prevent rickets. At the time, no one knew why cod liver oil was beneficial; they simply knew that something in it—like vitamin A or a similar fat-soluble chemical—was responsible.

It would take almost 15 years after Mellanby's discovery for cod liver oil supplementation to become common practice as a means of preventing and treating rickets. Cod liver oil became known as an antirachitic (antirickets) agent. While there may be enough vitamin D in cod liver oil to help prevent rickets, the blood levels obtained are not optimal for prevention of other diseases associated with vitamin D deficiency. Fortunately, mass supplementation of cod liver oil resulted in an overall improvement in children's health and child mortality subsequently plummeted.

Adolf Otto Reinhold Windaus (1876–1959), a German chemist who won the Nobel Prize in Chemistry in 1929, determined the chemical structures of vitamin D3 (cholecalciferol) and elicited the steps of its transformation from the beginning molecule of cholesterol. Interestingly, vitamin D had more in common with cholesterol and estrogen than with the other vitamins known at the time. However, since it was the fourth vitamin discovered, it was called vitamin D. For unknown reasons, he gave his patents to Merck and Bayer pharmaceuticals.

The discovery of vitamin D and its benefits helped lead the way to fortification of common food products so that disease prevention could occur.

Food Fortification

We can trace the importance of food fortification (Table 1) almost 2,500 years. In 400 BC, the Persian physician, Melanus, added iron to the wine of soldiers to increase their strength and give them a competitive edge against their enemies. In the 1930s, iodine, vitamin D, and B vitamins were routinely added to foods. Years later, folic acid fortified many grains and bread products.

Table 1. Nutrients that help prevent disease

Food Fortification and Disease Prevention
• Vitamin A prevents night blindness
• Vitamin B1 prevents beriberi (a nerve condition)
• Vitamin B6 prevents pellagra (triad of dementia, dermatitis and diarrhea)
• Vitamin C fortification prevents scurvy
• Vitamin D supplementation prevents rickets and many other diseases
• Iodine supplementation prevents goiter (enlarged thyroid gland)
• Folic Acid fortification prevents spina bifida (abnormal spinal closure of a newborn baby's spine)

In the 1940s, vitamin D routinely fortified milk and dairy products; as a result, rickets became a disease of the past—at least that is what people thought. Years later, orange juice also became fortified. Unfortunately, the low levels in milk (50 IU/8 oz) and orange juice (50 IU-100 IU/8 oz) prevent rickets, but don't provide the other health benefits of vitamin D that will be further discussed in this book.

Rickets Today

In 2003, Dr. Kumaravel Rajakumar (University of Pittsburgh School of Medicine) and Dr. Russell Chesney (The University of Tennessee Health Science Center) published articles in pediatric journals about the reemergence of rickets in North America. The cases involved African-American babies living in northern latitudes.

Today, rickets appears in babies who are predominantly breast-fed, as breast milk is traditionally seen as a poor source of vitamin D. The likely reason is that the breastfeeding moms are also deficient in vitamin D. Therefore, maternal vitamin D supplementation, especially in Hispanics and African-Americans, would be prudent in order to prevent the babies from being deficient. By supplementing, the mother's milk supply will become replete with vitamin D.

A 2008 article by Roni Caryn Rabin, published in the *New York Times*, discussed several cases of exclusively breast-fed infants who developed rickets, while others had severely low levels and were on the verge of rickets. The article also confirmed specialists' concerns about the re-emergence of rickets as more children avoid the outdoors and continue with their poor diets, which include sodas, juices, and less vitamin D-fortified milk.

In 2005, Judith Lazol, MD of Pittsburgh Children's Hospital, Pennsylvania, and her colleagues published a study in which they reviewed 58 cases of rickets in the United States from 1995 to 2005. The majority (81%) of these children were African-American; 14% were Arabic, and they were almost exclusively breast-fed.

In 2006, a study by Pamela Weisberg, RD (Maternal Child Nutrition Branch, Division of Nutrition and Physical Activity, Centers for Disease Control and Prevention, Atlanta) and colleagues studied 166 cases of rickets between 1986 and 2003. The data showed that 83% were African-American, and 96% of them were breast-fed.

The American Academy of Pediatrics recommends that children get at least 400 IU of vitamin D daily. Pregnant women are expected to get at least 400 IU daily, according to RDI guidelines. However, studies have shown that these levels are truly inadequate to achieve optimal blood levels. It is important that pregnant women and newborns have their vitamin D levels checked. I suspect over the next decade, physicians will start to order these tests with more frequency.

Why I Became Interested In Vitamin D

As a family medicine resident, I read an article in 2004 about vitamin D and its ability to help prevent falls in seniors. This study appeared in *American Family Physician*, a peer-reviewed journal of the American Academy of Family Physicians. I spoke of these findings with Dr. Wilfred Schach, an attending physician in my residency program. Dr. Schach is one of the most brilliant physicians and clinicians I have ever met. He had just turned 80 years old at the time and was as up-to-date on the medical literature as many of the young physicians he trained. He has excellent clinical skills and emphasized the importance of a complete and thorough physical exam. We live during a time when many physicians rely on the results of CT exams and ultrasounds instead of their own clinical impressions. Dr. Schach made sure that no future physicians whom he instructed let basic clinical medicine pass them by.

We debated the findings of this vitamin D study. Dr. Schach, a South African native, was aware of the side effects of vitamin D deficiency and assured me that since we were in Southern California—and therefore had plenty of sunlight—there was no need to waste money by checking patients' vitamin D levels. Unfortunately, most physicians living in Southern California and the rest of the United States share this sentiment. However, times are changing and I suspect that in the next 10 years, every physician in the United States and other industrialized countries will be ordering vitamin D levels as frequently as they order cholesterol and blood sugar tests.

In early 2009, I spoke with Dr. Schach, aka, the "Schach Attack" and was amazed to see that he remembered the vitamin D pathway in detail. I recommended he check his vitamin D level. He said he would.

By 2006, I was in private practice. I had a patient named Mary Farley (name changed). Mary was in her fifties and suffered miserably from fibromyalgia pain, which affected her every single day. Awakening in the morning and getting dressed for the day was an ordeal. Her days were "touch and go." She had difficulty making plans too far ahead, as she could never predict how she would feel. Over-the-counter pain medicines such as ibuprofen and acetaminophen (Tylenol®) were useless for her. She required narcotics and muscle relaxants in order to provide even minimal relief. Hydrocodone/acetaminophen (Vicodin®) and the muscle relaxant carisoprodol (Soma®) and, eventually, a narcotic pain patch could not control her pain. We tried everything known to help her get her life back. Even a consultation with a pain specialist was not productive in helping her control pain.

Being desperate for a solution and believing that one was out there, I did an online search for alternative treatments for fibromyalgia. I serendipitously came across an article on vitamin D deficiency and the symptoms associated with such deficiency. To my surprise, I came across a description in the online Merck Manual version and later confirmed it with my medical textbook of the same name. It stated:

"Vitamin D deficiency can cause muscle aches, muscle weakness, and bone pain at any age."

I then looked up the definition of fibromyalgia:

"Fibromyalgia is an increasingly recognized chronic pain illness that is characterized by widespread musculoskeletal aches, pain and stiffness, soft tissue tenderness, general fatigue, and sleep disturbances."

I could not help but wonder if my patients with fibromyalgia pain were simply suffering from a vitamin D deficiency. I remember thinking, "Certainly it could not be this simple." In 2006, I started to recommend that my patients with fibromyalgia take vitamin D2 (ergocalciferol) supplements. The U.S. recommended daily intake (RDI) is 600 IU of vitamin D for adults over 70 years of age, 400 units for those aged 51 to 70 years old, and 200 IU for those under 50. I aggressively recommended 2,000 IU for all my patients with fibromyalgia. In addition, I started to check their blood vitamin D levels.

To my surprise, 100% of my fibromyalgia patients were deficient. It seemed that those with the worst pain had the lowest levels. I could not believe my eyes. We live in Temecula, California—a desert located midway between Los Angeles and San Diego where the summer temperatures can reach 120°F (49 °C)in the shade. Surely, there is no shortage of sunlight. Then I realized that if people were like me and worked in an office all day, they could go the whole day with little to no sun exposure.

We start our days by getting into our garage-parked cars and driving around with our sunglasses on and our tinted windows—both of which block UV light. When we go to work or to the store, we look for the closest parking space. We get out, walk no more than 1 or 2 minutes, and then spend the rest of the day inside an enclosed building with closed windows and air conditioning. If we happen to go out to lunch, we may spend another 2 to 3 minutes in the sun. When the day is over, the sun is setting, and we arrive back home where it is dark. In other words, we get 3 to 5 minutes daily of direct sun exposure in one of the sunniest places on earth.

Unfortunately, when my patients with fibromyalgia came back in to follow up, they really did not notice any significant improvement in their pain symptoms after the vitamin D supplementation. I became disillusioned. Surely, there had to be a connection. It could not be a coincidence that those with the most pain also had the lowest levels of vitamin D in their blood. Mary stated that she felt a little better but I was not seeing the results I had hoped for. Others did not even feel this level of relief.

After starting my patients on vitamin D2 supplementation, I would wait 3 to 4 months before retesting their blood levels of vitamin D. I was shocked that their blood levels of vitamin D barely budged. At the time, I had tested over 20 patients with fibromyalgia and not one of them had a normal vitamin D blood level, that is, above 32 ng/ml (80 nmol/L). I waited another 3 months, and then retested—the results were the same. They were still deficient. Most were on 2,000 IU of vitamin D2 (ergocalciferol), an over-the-counter vitamin formulation. At 2,000 IU, they were taking 3 to 10 times the recommended dose. How could it be that they were still deficient?

The recommended daily intake set by the government is obviously inadequate. While the level recommended may prevent rickets, it is not even enough to get a person's blood level to normal 32 ng/ml (80 nmol/L) or greater. Note: Efforts are currently underway to encourage the government to increase this level.

In addition to vitamin D supplementation, I suggested that my patients increase their sunlight exposure, which is something a physician rarely recommends today. I am sure they thought my recommendations were peculiar. They came in for chronic pain symptoms and I was telling them to go outside and "work on their tan." I am certain my advice was rarely followed.

Haven't doctors, news programs, and magazine articles been preaching sun avoidance for the last two decades due to risk of skin cancers, which account for one million cases of cancer each year? (Fortunately, 95% of these are not life-threatening.) Doctors consistently urge patients to use sunscreen at all times. While this is smart, excessive use may prove to be dangerous to our health. I will discuss more about this later.

I was convinced I was onto something important. Although I have no proof, I am sure my colleagues were hoping I would take over care of their fibromyalgia patients, as it is difficult to help them become pain-free.

At first, my colleagues likely thought I was crazy. Initially I, too, started to wonder whether I was sane. Pregabalin (Lyrica®) was being marketed as the first FDA-approved medicine for fibromyalgia and I was recommending vitamin D. I even shared my information with the Lyrica drug reps but found little interest. Ironically, a patient who worked as a drug rep for another product line came in to see me with clinical signs of fibromyalgia. I checked her blood levels of vitamin D and she was deficient. I recommended supplementation and, fortunately, her pain symptoms improved. Years later, she is still pain free.

As my research continued, I started to come across articles that showed that vitamin D could help prevent and treat many other diseases that afflict people. Table 2 is a list of common diseases more prevalent in those with lower levels of vitamin D in their blood. I will discuss each in more detail throughout the book.

Table 2. Diseases and conditions associated with low vitamin D levels

Diseases and Conditions Associated with Low Vitamin D blood levels	
• Osteopenia	• Overweight
• Osteoporosis	• Colon cancer
• Falls	• Prostate cancer
• Chronic pain	• Breast cancer
• Fibromyalgia	• Ovarian cancer
• Heart disease	• Cervical cancer
• High blood pressure	• Pancreatic cancer
• Type I diabetes	• Multiple sclerosis
• Type II diabetes	• Melanoma
• Obesity	• Psoriasis

Biochemistry of Vitamin D

Vitamin D comes in two forms: vitamin D2 (ergocalciferol) and vitamin D3 (cholecalciferol). Most references in this book to vitamin D refer to vitamin D3 and not vitamin D2. Vitamin D2 and D3 are not really vitamins in the classic sense, but are actually steroid-like molecules—not the type of steroid that a bodybuilder takes to bulk up, but the kind that your body makes to help with stressful situations. The vitamin D (Figure 4) structure has more in common with cortisol, estrogen (the female hormone), and testosterone (the male hormone) than with vitamin C or vitamin E.

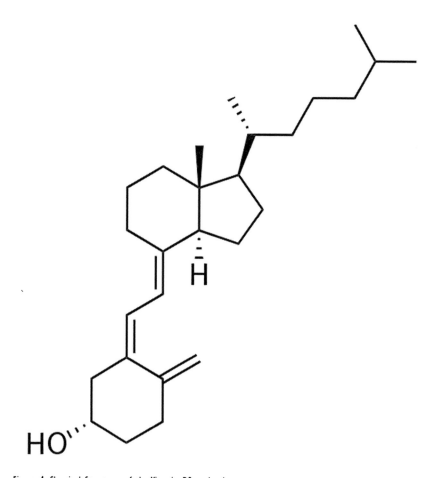

Figure 4. Chemical Structures of the Vitamin D3 molecule.

Vitamin D is manufactured when UVB (ultraviolet B) light waves (290 to 320 nm) from the sun combine with a substance in the skin, provitamin D3 (7-dehydrocholesterol, or 7DHC), a "cousin" of the cholesterol molecule found in the skin. The result is the formation of previtamin D3, which is transformed to the more stable molecule, vitamin D3 (cholecalciferol). Vitamin D3 travels through the blood and ultimately to the liver where it is converted to 25-hydroxyvitamin D, by an enzyme called 25-hydroxylase. The 25-hydroxyvitamin D (Vitamin D 25-OH) then travels to the kidneys and other tissues in the body where it becomes vitamin D 1,25 OH after it reacts with the 1-alpha hydroxylase enzymes. It is this molecule (1,25 hydroxy-vitamin) that exerts its health benefits on our bodies.

> # Provitamin D3 (7-DHC) → Previtamin D3 → Vitamin D3 →25 hydroxy-vitamin D→ 1,25 hydroxy-vitamin D (the form which has effects on organs)

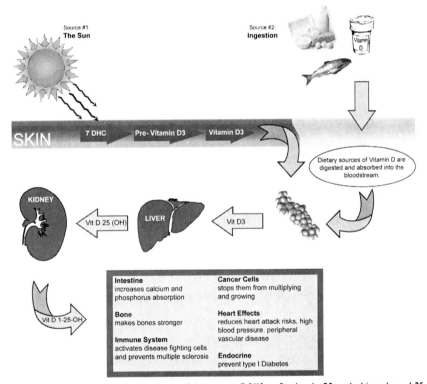

Figure: 5. Vitamin D Pathway showing how sunlight converts 7-DHC to Previtamin D3, and ultimately to 1,25 hydroxyvitamin D, the form which has positive effects on our health. Image illlustrated by Jennifer M. Clare.

Over the years, studies have shown that other organs such as the colon, prostate, and muscles also contain the ability to use vitamin D 25-OH and convert it to the active form. In addition, these organs have vitamin D receptors. This research has helped scientists realize the health benefits and cancer fighting properties of vitamin D.

Vitamin D, when in the blood in sufficient quantities, helps facilitate the absorption of calcium and phosphorus through the intestinal wall and into the bloodstream. This helps maintain a balance of these very important minerals.

In 1937, Dr. Ragnar Nicolaysen from The Nutritional Laboratory, University of Cambridge and Medical Research Council, discovered that vitamin D was required for calcium absorption in the gut. When vitamin D levels are deficient, calcium is not optimally absorbed. As a result, our bodies try to find a source of calcium somewhere else in the body. Any ideas where our body is hiding calcium? Our bones! However, calcium in our bones does not simply jump out of our bones into our blood; it needs help.

When our vitamin D levels are low, the body makes a hormone called PTH (parathyroid hormone) that subsequently mobilizes calcium from the skeletal bones and releases it into the bloodstream. You can imagine that, if this continues to occur year after year, bones become thinner and thinner, ultimately leading to osteomalacia, osteopenia (thin bones), and eventually osteoporosis. When a person with weak bones falls, he or she is at high risk of bone fractures and the associated complications.

Secondary hyperparathyroidism, the medical condition associated with a high level of PTH in the blood, is a condition associated with osteopenia and osteoporosis. I will discuss these conditions in more detail later in the book.

Genes, Genetic Code, and Vitamin D Receptors

In 2003, the Human Genome Project, a decade-long project of mapping out the human genetic code, was completed. Scientists were able to "decode" human chromosomes and determine the sequence of our genes. In essence, they deciphered the very blueprint of what makes us human.

This was an amazing discovery and occurred just 50 years after Francis Crick and James Watson discovered the DNA structure (Figure 6). Their findings appeared in the scientific journal *Nature* in April, 1953. At the time, they knew they were onto something big, but did not really understand the significance of their discovery. In the one-page article, they wrote, "This structure has novel features which are of considerable biological interest."

26

Watson and Crick, along with Maurice Wilkins, earned the Noble Prize for their shared discovery, a discovery that would revolutionize science for generations to come.

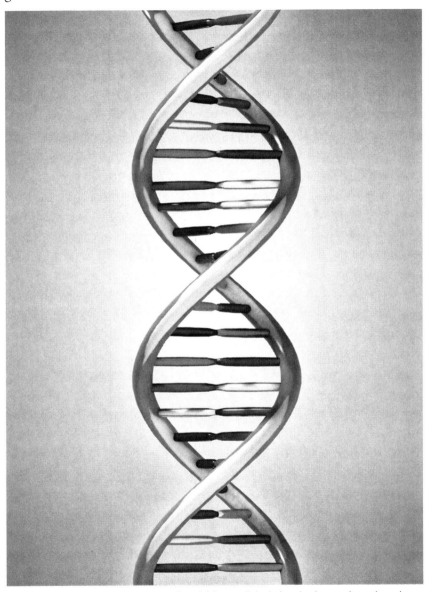

Figure 6. DNA double helix structure consists of 4 bases called adenine, thymine, guanine and cytosine. (BigStockPhoto.com © Tony Sanchez)

Each healthy human has 46 total chromosomes, 23 from Mom and 23 from Dad. To study chromosomes, scientists numbered them 1 through 22, plus the X and Y chromosomes, which determine our sex. These chromosomes consist of DNA (deoxyribonucleic acid), our genetic "instruction manual." The DNA consists of four chemical "bases" called guanine, cytosine, thymine, and adenine. This is how we pass our genetic information on to our children and grandchildren, which explains why one may have Grandma's eyes but Mom's nose. According to the National Institutes of Health (NIH) publication entitled, *What is a Genome?*, each human has about 20,500 genes—which makes us unique. Interestingly, a grain of rice has up to 55,000 genes, while a dog about 19,000 genes. I assume this was done to keep us humble as a species—an example of celestial comedy.

Our genes determine quite a bit about us. They encode the instructions for hair color, hair texture, eye color, skin color, and whether or not one is at risk for certain diseases, such as breast cancer. Genes determine whether a person will be bald at 40 or have a full head of hair at 70. In addition, the genes encode how long one will live.

Fortunately, most genes don't just turn on or off by themselves. They need to be activated. Within you, you have the power to control your genes. You heard me right! The choices you and I make every day can ultimately decide whether we turn on our disease-causing genes or turn on our healthy longevity disease-free genes. As Wes Youngberg, MPH, DrPH, a founding director for the American College of Lifestyle Medicine and Director of the Rancho Wellness Center in Temecula, CA states, "Our genes are not our destiny." This is an important fact to realize. To blame one's diabetes or high blood pressure on family medical history is not an excuse.

Dr. Madrid, how do I turn on my healthy genes and turn off my disease causing genes? We can do this if we improve our diet, eat more whole foods, and consume generous servings of fruits and vegetables that don't have pesticides on them. In addition, we need to minimize environmental exposure to chemicals and stop heating foods in plastic containers. Chemicals found in plastics, like bisphenol A (BPA), can negatively affect our hormones, which ultimately can affect our longevity. Increasing exercise and minimizing stress can also have beneficial effects on our genes, turning on life-promoting genes and turning off the disease-causing genes.

Certain minerals, vitamins and herbal adaptogens, when present in adequate concentrations, can help prevent diseases. This has turned out to be the case for vitamin D. When our bodies have optimal vitamin D, they can literally turn off certain cancer cells by influencing our DNA. This is evident in several studies that showed those with more vitamin D in their blood had a 12% (Michos 2007) to 22% (Trivedi 2003) reduction in all causes of mortality. In other words, those with more vitamin D in their blood were 12% to 22% less likely to die from any cause.

> ## "Those with more vitamin D in their blood were 12–22% less likely to die from any cause."

A vitamin D molecule acts like a key, binding to a vitamin D receptor (VDR), or lock. The result is that the gene is turned on like a key opens a door. Researchers have determined that the genes that make vitamin D receptors are chromosome 12. A vitamin D receptor is unique for vitamin D (just as a key is specific for a particular lock) and allows us to realize the health benefits of it. Initially, scientists thought that vitamin D acted only on the bones, but years of research show that vitamin D also affects every other tissue and cell. The vitamin D receptor is an important part of the cell, affecting cell behavior. In addition, vitamin D influences cellular pathways. Specifically, the vitamin D molecule has the ability to turn genes on or off. When the cells get the appropriate message, the cells create proteins that can influence our health in positive ways. For example, when cancer cells are given adequate vitamin D, they are given a signal to "self destruct," a term scientists call *apoptosis*.

Scientists have discovered that the following tissues and organs have vitamin D receptors, meaning vitamin D needs to be present in adequate concentrations for these parts of the body to function normally.

- Adrenal glands
- Bones
- Bone marrow
- Brain
- Breast Tissue

- Cartilage surfaces
- Colon (Large Intestine)
- Fat cells
- Kidneys
- Liver
- Lung Tissue
- Lymphocytes
- Muscle tissues
- Ovaries
- Pancreas cells (which make insulin)
- Parathyroid gland
- Parotid gland
- Pituitary glands
- Prostate Gland
- Skin
- Small Intestine
- Stomach Tissue
- Testicles
- Thyroid Gland
- Uterus

Imagine if a person had more vitamin D receptors within his or her cells. The person with more receptors could benefit from vitamin D at lower blood levels than a person with fewer receptors.

Scientists have discovered vitamin D genes and have named them FokI, ApaI, TaqI, Cdx2, and BsmI. A study reported in the *Annals of Internal Medicine* and conducted by Dr. Andre Uitterlinden (Erasmus University School of Medicine, The Netherlands) and colleagues showed that those with the Cdx2 gene polymorphism had up to a 13% risk reduction in vertebral fractures. This indicates that some people may be genetically protected from fracturing their bones.

Studies also show that certain forms of vitamin D act on nuclear VDRs to signal cells on a biochemical level. Effects include cell regulation, apoptosis (cell destruction, especially bad ones like cancer), and generation of cytokines, which have antimicrobial effects.

A study by Wendy Chen, MD, MPH (Dana Farber Cancer Institute, Boston, USA), concluded that VDRs may be a mediator of breast cancer risk and could represent a target for breast cancer prevention. The good news is that this pathway likely affects all cancers so additional research on vitamin D receptors could prove to be the holy grail of cancer treatment. More research is required on this growing field of science and genetics.

Pharmaceutical companies are quickly working on vitamin D analogues to patent for cancer treatment. These are, in essence, "copycat" vitamin D molecules that they hope will treat and prevent cancer. Why not use regular vitamin D? Drug companies hope they can improve on what nature has already provided. Also, since vitamin D itself cannot be patented, there is virtually no money to be made in the mass marketing and distribution of it. However, it's OK with me if drug companies don't make billions at our expense. The goal is to reduce human suffering and disease with the least expensive method possible.

How Common Is Vitamin D Deficiency?

When I suggest to patients that we check their vitamin D levels, as they are probably deficient, they usually deny this possibility. I frequently hear statements such as, "I am out in the sun a lot, I am sure I am fine," or "No need to check, Doc, I take a calcium supplement and it has vitamin D in it." I then tell my patient that even I was deficient in vitamin D when I had my vitamin D level checked. I also take a multivitamin daily, which has 800 IU of vitamin D. This had minimal impact on my blood levels.

In the last several years, physicians and scientists have started to realize the numerous health benefits that vitamin D, when optimized, has to offer and the public health consequences of a blood vitamin D deficiency.

In medical school, students learn that a vitamin D deficiency causes rickets. However, since rickets is rarely seen by physicians in the U.S., Europe, or other developed countries, it is assumed that vitamin D deficiency is nonexistent, especially since milk, orange juice, and other foods are often fortified with vitamin D. It now appears that rickets is only the beginning and that patients need higher levels to prevent a myriad of other conditions.

Hundreds of studies have appeared in leading medical journals showing that vitamin D deficiency is a worldwide epidemic. Americans are not the only ones. Europeans, Irish, Australians, British, Saudis, Asian-Indians, and many others are all short of the sunshine vitamin. Studies have shown that vitamin D deficiencies affect the majority of all populations studied.

While a vitamin D level above 12 ng/ml (30 nmol/L) can prevent rickets, we need levels above 32 ng/ml to keep bones strong, and levels as high as 50 ng/ml (125 nmol/L) to reduce the incidence of colon cancer by up to 60%. Identification of this deficiency and appropriate treatment will have global implications. Billions of people will benefit from this simple, inexpensive treatment.

Prior to my research a few years ago and routine screening for vitamin D deficiency, I didn't think anyone in Southern California was deficient in the sunshine vitamin. However, our medical practice has since diagnosed thousands of patients with vitamin D deficiency, or about 80% of all patients tested. Our findings are similar to other studies and their reporting of vitamin D deficiencies.

Vitamin D deficiency was known to be a problem in the 1980s. One report by Dr. Charlotte Egsmose published in *Age and Ageing* in 1987, described a study of 94 seniors in a long-stay nursing home. Their average vitamin D blood levels were 24 ng/ml (60 nmol/L). In addition, half of the people in the study had levels under 5ng/ml (12.5 nmol/L). The authors of that study concluded that daily vitamin D supplementation was indicated for elderly people in nursing homes. None had normal vitamin D levels above 32 ng/ml (80 nmol/L).

Interestingly, almost 25 years later, most physicians still don't check blood levels for vitamin D, nor do they recommend vitamin D supplementation for their senior citizen patients. Fortunately, with all the research published in the last 5 years demonstrating the health benefits of vitamin D, more and more physicians are starting to check their patients' vitamin D blood levels.

It is my hope that, with this book, more people will ask their doctors to check their vitamin D levels. Personally, I recommend all my seniors take vitamin D supplementation. I check their blood levels regularly to ensure that they are getting the correct dose.

Several factors can lead to vitamin D deficiency in all ages including obesity, lack of sun exposure, darker pigment, use of sunscreen, wearing long sleeves and hats, tinted auto windows, air pollution, cloudy days, geographical location, and the season. As Dr. John Cannell, Vitamin D Council Executive Director, points out in a review article on vitamin D deficiency, African-Americans, the obese, and the elderly are at additional risk.

In our natural state, humans spend most of the time outdoors, working the fields, gardening, gathering food, and building shelter. It has only been in the last several hundred years that we have become predominantly an indoor species. According to a study by Reinhold Vieth, PhD (Director of the Bone and Mineral Laboratory at the University of Toronto), most people who spend the majority of time outdoors have a vitamin D blood level of 50-70 ng/ml (125-175 nmol/L). Further, most studies show that we should strive for this range.

Risk factors for vitamin D deficiency include the following:

- Obesity
- Lack of sun exposure
- Darker pigment
- Age >60
- Use of sunscreen
- Wearing long sleeves and hats
- Air pollution
- Cloudy days
- Geographical location
- Winter and Spring Seasons
- Tinted automobile windows

Children and Vitamin D Deficiency

Children are at high risk for vitamin D deficiency. This risk starts when a baby is developing in his/her mother's uterus and continues throughout adolescence. Physicians and patients alike should suspect a vitamin D deficiency. When present, it can lead to stunted growth, weak bones, and increased risk of osteoporosis later in life. Even if your child drinks milk every day, s/he is still at risk for vitamin D deficiency, as each glass of milk has between 50 IU to 100 IU of vitamin D. A 2008 report by Serena Gordon published in the *Washington Post* stated: "At least 40% of American infants and toddlers aren't getting enough vitamin D, according to researchers from Children's Hospital in Boston."

Many physicians are starting to recognize that this is a serious problem. I challenge the American Academy of Pediatrics (AAP) to come out with a position statement recommending routine vitamin D screening for all children, starting at birth. In addition, the American Academy of Family Physicians needs to come out with a similar position.

In October 2008, the AAP recommended doubling the recommended dose of vitamin D from 200 IU/day to 400 IU/day, but this does not go far enough, in my opinion, and in the opinions of many others who research vitamin D. If a child were relying on milk to provide this requirement, the child would need to drink eight 4- to 8-ounce glasses of milk daily to get this amount of vitamin D. Most family doctors and pediatricians recommend that children not drink more than 24 ounces of milk per day. As mentioned earlier, my multivitamin had 800 IU of vitamin D and my blood levels were deficient.

Most children will need a dose higher than 400 IU daily—exactly how much can be determined only through a blood test. In the meantime, physicians should consider adding a vitamin D testing to the 1-year hemoglobin test or the 2- to 4-year cholesterol test that is now recommended for some children.

The AAP has boldly recommended routine cholesterol screening for at-risk children starting at 2 years and possible cholesterol drugs for those children over age 8 with high cholesterol and other risk factors. Some may argue that if vitamin D pills cost $60/month, there would be a marketing budget available to help promote the product and large scale consumption. Fortunately for the consumer, the cost is closer to $3 to $5 per month or less.

Infants and toddlers are not the only ones who are deficient; teenagers also are at high risk of vitamin D deficiency.

In 2008, a study reported by Mary Brophy Marcus in *USA Today* showed that 42% of teenagers were deficient in vitamin D. Another study by Dr. Catherine Gordon (Children's Hospital, Boston, USA) concluded, "Vitamin D deficiency was present in many U.S. adolescents in this...sample. The prevalence was highest in African-American teenagers and during winter, although the problem seems to be common across sex, season, and ethnicity."

A separate study published in 2000 by Grace Wyshak, PhD (Harvard School of Public Health), in the *Archives of Pediatrics and Adolescent Medicine*, showed that urban high school girls who reported themselves as being physically active and who consumed carbonated beverages (soda pop) were 3 to 5 times more likely to have bone fractures than those who did not consume carbonated beverages. It is likely that a low vitamin D status, in addition to low calcium intake due to soda replacing milk, contributed to their overall poor bone strength and increased fracture risk.

The take-home message here is that physicians need to screen all children and teenagers for vitamin D deficiency. We need to encourage young people to go outside more, ride their bikes, skateboards, and play ball at the park. Using sunscreen to prevent sunburns is important but balancing that with adequate sun exposure is crucial. We need to limit the amount of time spent watching television, playing video games, and drinking sugary drinks and other sweetened, carbonated beverages.

A rule of thumb that I use for my own children is that they should spend more time playing outside and reading books than watching TV or playing video games.

Vitamin D Deficiency and Pregnancy

The demands on a woman's body during pregnancy are enormous. During pregnancy, many hormonal changes take place and various stresses affect her body. Evidence shows that pregnant women are just as likely to be deficient in vitamin D as anyone else. However, with the nutritional demands of a growing baby, this deficiency can lead to poor bone development in the young child. If present, it is important to identify the deficiency.

During pregnancy, a woman's recommended daily intake (RDI) levels for many nutrients increase to help meet the increased demands. This includes increased demand for calcium and iron. However, the American College of Obstetricians and Gynecology currently does not have specific recommendations beyond the RDI for vitamin D. However, if vitamin D levels were checked in most pregnant women, I am certain they would be just as deficient as in nonpregnant women.

A 2005 study published in the *American Journal of Clinical Nutrition* by Alok Sachan, PhD (Department of Endocrinology, Sanjay Gandhi Postgraduate Institute of Medical Sciences), and colleagues showed that 84% of pregnant women in India were vitamin D deficient. Their newborn babies were also deficient.

A 2007 report in *Clinical Pediatrics* of American women showed that 50% of postpartum mothers and 65% of their newborn infants had severe vitamin D deficiency, with blood levels less than 12 ng/ml (30 nmol/l). This level is low enough to cause rickets.

A 2006 study by Kassim Javaid, BSMed Sci, PhD (School of Medicine, University of Southampton, Southampton, UK), published in *The Lancet* concluded:

> Maternal vitamin D insufficiency is common during pregnancy and is associated with reduced bone-mineral (weak bones)…in the offspring during childhood ….Vitamin D supplementation of pregnant women, especially during winter months, could lead to long-lasting reductions in the risk of osteoporotic fracture in their offspring.

In other words, when pregnant moms are vitamin D deficient—as were 49% of the women in this study—their children are at risk of weaker bones and, ultimately for developing osteoporosis as adults. The good news is that vitamin D supplementation can prevent this. The amount of vitamin D in prenatal vitamins is commonly insufficient.

In 2008, *Science Daily* reported on a study from University of Manitoba, Winnipeg, Canada. The results showed that women with vitamin D deficiency during pregnancy also placed their children at risk for poor tooth development and tooth decay.

Anne Merewood, MPH (Boston University), and colleagues published a study in the *Journal of Clinical Endocrinology & Metabolism* in 2008. They enrolled 253 pregnant women in their study. Of these, 38 women had a Cesarean section. Further analysis showed that 28% of the women with a vitamin D level less than 15 ng/ml (37.5 nmol/L) had a Cesarean section, compared to 14% of women who had levels above 15 ng/ml (37.5 nmol/L). When further analysis was done that factored race, alcohol use, education, and health insurance, the researchers concluded "women with vitamin D blood levels less than 15 ng/ml (37.5 nmol/L) were almost 4 times more likely to have a Cesarean section than women with vitamin D levels above 15 ng/ml (37.5 nmol/L).

Lastly, a separate study from the United Kingdom, published in the *British Journal of Gynaecology* in 2002, concluded that, "In view of the high incidence of subnormal vitamin D levels in women from ethnic minorities, we recommend…[vitamin D] screening of these women in early pregnancy, with subsequent supplementation where indicated."

I am certain that, within the next few years, Obstetricians will start to check vitamin D levels with routine prenatal labs. In the meantime, all pregnant women should ask their obstetricians or family physician to check their vitamin D levels and then begin supplementation with at least 2,000 IU of vitamin D daily, or more, after discussing the blood test results with their physicians. Prenatal vitamins have only between 400 to 800 IU of vitamin D. Currently, I am unaware of studies suggesting that higher levels pose any harm to a growing baby. If there were a known harm, doctors would advise pregnant women to avoid the sun to prevent too much vitamin D from being generated. Few doctors are aware of vitamin D deficiency during pregnancy and its potential harms. Readers should share the information in this book with their ob-gyns.

Vitamin D Deficiency in African-Americans

Those with darker pigment are at increased risk of vitamin D deficiency when compared to those with lighter skin. As a result, it is crucial that all African-Americans and others of African descent have their vitamin D blood levels checked. This is especially important for anyone who has fewer than 1 hour of optimal sunlight exposure each day.

Ultraviolet light (UV-B) from the sun reacts with a substance in the skin to form vitamin D. Since skin melanin, the protein responsible for pigment, acts as a natural sunscreen, those with darker skin require about 6 times more exposure in the sun compared to a lighter-skinned person in order to produce the same amount of vitamin D. Vitamin D deficiency is common in over 75% of African-Americans.

While basal cell and squamous cell cancers are unlikely in those of African descent, melanomas—especially on the soles, palms, and fingernail beds—can occur in this population. In addition, we know that melanoma is more deadly in African-Americans. Therefore, routine skin checks should be part of yearly physicals. If your doctor does not do this, please request it. Numerous studies have shown that African-Americans have lower serum vitamin D levels on a larger scale when compared to those with lighter skin.

However, no one is immune from vitamin D deficiency. Interestingly, having adequate vitamin D actually protects against many cancers, including melanoma. I will discuss this more in the melanoma section.

A study by Marian Hannan, MPH, DSc (Beth Israel Deaconess Medical Center and associate professor at Harvard Medical School) of 1,114 people showed that African-Americans and Hispanics are more likely to be vitamin D deficient when compared to whites. This is due to their increased skin pigmentation. Not surprisingly, the groups with darker pigment also suffer more from various diseases, even when access to health-care services and medicines are the same.

An additional study by Elizabeth Jacobs, PhD (Assistant Professor at the University of Arizona), and colleagues showed at least 45–55% of African-Americans are deficient in vitamin D, while up to 37% of Hispanics are. However, this study used 20 ng/ml (50 nmol/L), instead of 32 ng/ml (80 nmol/L), as a reference range for normal, so the results underestimate the true deficiency rate.

A study published in *The Journal of Nutrition* by Susan S. Harris, DSc (Boston University School of Public Health), concluded:

A high percentage of American blacks have suboptimal blood levels of 25(OH)D and levels that are well below those of American whites. Poor vitamin D status may increase the risk of blacks as well as others for osteoporosis, cardiovascular disease, cancers, diabetes, and other serious chronic conditions.

A study by Dr. Catherine Gordon, Children's Hospital, Boston, concluded that, "Vitamin D deficiency was present in many US adolescents in this urban clinic-based sample...[and] was highest in African American teenagers."

A second study by Susan S. Harris, DSc (Boston University School of Public Health), of people aged 64 to 100, showed that 73% of the African-Americans had vitamin D concentrations less than 20 ng/ml (50 nmol/L). Since the number we now consider normal is above 32 ng/ml (80 nmol/L), 73% underestimates the true number of people who are deficient. My experience suggests that the number is closer to 90%. This led the authors of the study to conclude that, "elderly individuals who live in northern areas, particularly African-Americans, should be strongly encouraged to increase their vitamin D intake, especially in winter."

Another study by Dr. Richard D. Semba, Johns Hopkins University School of Medicine, and colleagues was published in the *American Journal of Clinical Nutrition*. Researchers concluded that, "Vitamin D deficiency, a preventable disorder, is a common and important public health problem... black women are at higher risk than are white women."

> **"Vitamin D deficiency may be the main reason that colon cancer, prostate cancer, breast cancer, high blood pressure, strokes, and heart disease affect African-Americans to a higher degree..."**

Many scientists, including myself, believe that high vitamin D deficiency rates may be the main reason that colon cancer, prostate cancer, breast cancer, high blood pressure, strokes, and heart disease affect African-Americans to a higher degree than they affect those with lighter skin. In addition, once diagnosed, the prognosis is poorer. Vitamin D deficiency may even contribute to the poor survival rate from melanoma among African-Americans, which is half that of whites. Even when the studies control for health insurance coverage, socioeconomic status, and access to quality health care and treatment, those with darker skin and ultimately, lower vitamin D levels, have poorer outcomes.

Edward Giovannucci, MD, ScD (Harvard School of Public Health), and colleagues conducted a study that was published in 2006. They concluded, "Our results suggest that the high frequency of hypovitaminosis D (low vitamin D in the blood) in Blacks may be an important, and easily modifiable, contributor to their higher risk of cancer incidence and mortality."

My recommendation is that all African-Americans, Hispanics, Native Americans, and any other person of color, have their serum vitamin D level checked. It is important to call your doctor today and make an appointment to be seen. Ensuring adequate vitamin D supplementation will be one of the most important things you can do to improve your longevity and wellness. If you have already been diagnosed with any of the above conditions, optimizing your vitamin D levels can help manage your disease and improve your chance of survival.

It is important that you work closely with your doctor to do so. I recommend you attempt to achieve a vitamin D blood level above 50 ng/ml (125 nmol/L) for optimal health. It would not be uncommon to need doses up to 5,000 IU daily to achieve this level.

Vitamin D Deficiency in "Healthy" Adults

By this point, you may be saying, "I am not a child, pregnant, or African-American. Certainly I am not at risk—correct, Dr. Madrid?" WRONG!

Vitamin D deficiency is not something that affects only children or those with darker skin—it can affect every adult, no matter what background, socioeconomic status, race, or religion. Vitamin D deficiency affects those from 18 to 65, from every background, just as frequently as it affects those under 18 or over 65.

Dr. Linda B. White wrote in her *Mother Earth News* article that 81% of the British adults tested had vitamin D levels below 30 ng/ml (75 nmol/L) during the winter and spring, while 60% were deficient during the summer and fall.

In 2006, Elizabeth Jacobs, PhD (University of Arizona), showed that adults in Arizona, a state with the most sunshine, also suffered from vitamin D deficiency. She included 637 people in the study and only 22.7% had levels above 30 ng/ml (75 nmol/L). Among them, 77% were overall deficient. In other words, more than three out of four people were deficient. In addition, 2% of the population studied had levels less than 10 ng/ml (25 nmol/L), a level low enough to cause rickets.

In 2002, Michael Holick, MD, PhD (Professor of Medicine at Boston University), cited a number of studies that demonstrated vitamin D deficiency as high as 36% in white men and women in Boston and as high as 42% in African-American women. However, most of these studies underestimate the true deficiency status, as the researchers considered levels of 15 ng/ml (37.5 nmol/L) to be normal. Again, today, we define normal as anything above 32 ng/ml (80 nmol/L).

A 2000 study published in the *Journal of Internal Medicine*, by Henning Glerup, MD, PhD (University Hospital of Aarhus, Denmark), compared veiled Muslim women of Arab descent, who lived in Denmark to nonveiled Danish women. The veiled women were severely deficient when compared with Danish women who were not veiled, although, both groups were deficient. The study went on to conclude:

> Severe vitamin D deficiency is prevalent amongst sunlight-deprived individuals living in Denmark. In veiled Arab women, vitamin D deficiency is the result of a combination of limitations in sunlight exposure and a low oral intake of vitamin D. The oral intake of vitamin D amongst veiled ethnic Danish Moslems was, however, very high, at 13.53 μg (approximately 600 IU/day), but they were still vitamin D-deficient. Our results suggest that the daily oral intake of vitamin D in sunlight-deprived individuals should exceed 600 IU; most probably it should be 1,000 IU per day to secure a normal level of vitamin D in the blood. This finding is in contrast with the commonly used RDI (recommended daily intake) for adults in Europe: 200 IU per day.

Overall, people in Europe tend to be more deficient than people in the U.S., and people who live in more northern latitudes are more deficient than those living closer to the equator.

The main point is that all women, men, and children need to have their vitamin D blood levels checked. Call your physician today and schedule an appointment for a vitamin D blood test. As you will see in the following chapters, one should strive to have vitamin D levels greater than 50 ng/ml (125 nmol/L) for optimal bone health and cancer prevention. While the study from Denmark recommends at least 1,000 IU daily of vitamin D, my experience shows that this is too low for most people to be at optimal levels. I and most vitamin D experts from the vitamin D council recommend a minimal intake of 2,000 IU daily. However, many will need even a higher dose if their blood levels are not adequate.

Vitamin D Deficiency and Obesity

A person is considered obese if they have a body mass index (BMI) above 30 or are 30 pounds overweight. Obesity affects about one in four people in the U.S. Worldwide, the obesity epidemic has affected both adults and children, to our detriment, and the number of overweight and obese people is increasing at alarming rates, posing a serious threat to human health and longevity.

The introduction of processed foods and food additives in the 1970s, such as high fructose corn syrup (HFCS) and monosodium glutamate (MSG) has had catastrophic results. These additives, in combination with decreased physical activity, increased television viewing, and video game playing, are largely to blame for obesity. Studies have shown that foods that contain both HFCS and MSG put people at increased risk for obesity. An article in *Science Daily* (2008) reported that HFCS is abundant in sweetened beverages while MSG use diminishes the brain's ability to receive an "I AM FULL—STOP EATING" message. The result is overeating sugary foods without a signal to stop. So perhaps eating artificial sweeteners is the answer, right? Unfortunately not. Aspartame (NutraSweet), which is found in over 5,000 products, including diet beverages and foods, actually stimulates appetite, leading to increased calorie consumption.

> ## "The number of children between 6 and 11 years of age who are obese has almost tripled in the last 20 years—going from 6.5% in the 1980s to 17% today"

According to the Center for Disease Control (CDC), the number of children between 6 and 11 years of age who are obese has almost tripled in the last 20 years—going from 6.5% in the 1980s to 17% today (Figure 7). In adolescents aged 12 to 19 years, the rate has more than tripled, from 5% to 17%. In the 1980s and before, most classrooms in America had at least 1 or maybe 2 obese children, out of a class of 30 children. Today, the numbers are quite different. It is now common to see 5 or 6 obese children in a class of 30. This fact is tragic and outright dangerous for our survival.

Each of these overweight children is at very high risk for diabetes, high cholesterol, high blood pressure, elevated C reactive protein (CRP), kidney disease, cancer, and ultimately heart attacks. These at-risk children actually have a high likelihood of dying at a younger age than their parents. A 2005 *New York Times* article by Pam Belluck reported that if the trend continues, and it is, the current generation of children will have a *5- to 7-year shorter lifespan than their parents*. Furthermore, most parents of overweight and obese children don't consider their children as such, usually because the parents are also overweight.

Next time your child has a physical examination, ask your doctor to measure your child's BMI and show you where your child is on the BMI curve. BMI measurement differs for children and adults. Your child will be considered *normal weight, overweight, or obese*. If overweight or obese, ask for a referral to a nutritionist and get the family exercising immediately. Your child's health depends on it.

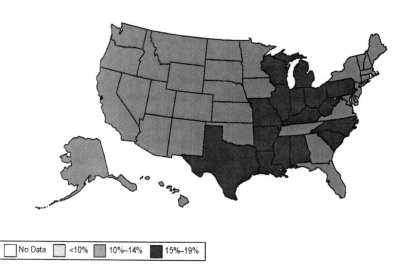

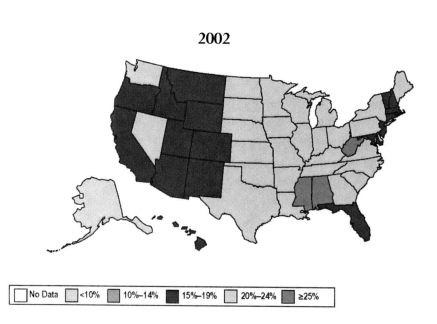

2007

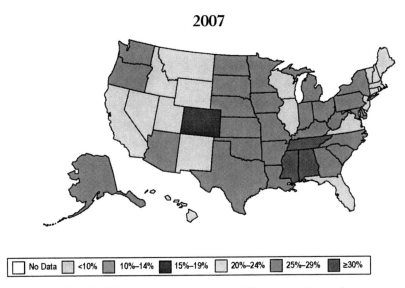

Figure 7. CDC Maps showing percentage of the U.S population who are obese (BMI>30) during years 1994, 2002 and 2007.

Children are not the only ones at risk. Nationally, over 25% of adults are considered obese (BMI >30) and another 30% are overweight (BMI 25.1-30). Being overweight or obese is a risk factor for many diseases and conditions, including vitamin D deficiency. This is because vitamin D is fat-soluble, meaning vitamin D in the blood is absorbed by fat cells.

As a result, studies consistently show that vitamin D deficiency is extremely common among the obese, and that vitamin D blood levels are 57% lower in obese people when compared to non-obese people. Estimates show that more than 90% of people who are obese are vitamin D deficient according to a study published by Jacobo Wortsman, MD (Southern Illinois University School of Medicine), in the *American Journal of Clinical Nutrition*.

The tendency for overweight and obese people to be vitamin D deficient likely contributes, in part, to their increased risk for diabetes, high blood pressure, and most cancers. Poor diet and lack of physical activities also are risk factors.

Simply put, if you have a bigger belly than you would like, you need to have your blood vitamin D level checked. Even if you like your big belly, you should still have your blood tested. Chances are you are deficient and need to work on elevating your levels. I recommend increased sunlight exposure and starting with 2,000 IU of vitamin D supplementation. After 3 months, you should ask your doctor to recheck your blood level. Achieving a vitamin D level above 50 ng/ml (125 nmol/L) should be the goal.

If you are overweight or obese, I strongly recommend that you see a certified nutritionist or trainer to get your weight to a healthier level. Consult with your physician first to ensure you can safely begin an exercise routine. This act alone will provide you with many more quality years of life and prevent many diseases.

Vitamin D Deficiency in Senior Citizens

The *golden years* are supposed to be the time when people enjoy the fruits of their years labored. This is when people who have worked their whole lives raising children, paying a mortgage, and giving unselfishly to others finally have time to themselves.

Many have an image of Grandma and Grandpa getting up in the morning, drinking their cups of coffee or green tea, reading the paper, and taking a morning walk—smelling the roses on the way. Perhaps they will go on a cruise or two or visit a casino. Why? Because this is what senior citizens are supposed to do—or is it?

Unfortunately, for many seniors, life is not this simple and enjoyable. Many retired individuals find it hard to live off a fixed income or to re-enter the work force. Many pensions are in danger as companies that were, at one time, the fabric of America are in jeopardy of closing their doors. Social security payments are not keeping up with inflation and its survival is in question.

In addition, many seniors are taking care of grandchildren while trying to manage their chronic diseases. Attending doctor appointments regularly can be quite expensive and co-pays can quickly add up. For many, weak muscles and disease have made the golden years challenging and not as fulfilling as they could be.

A patient came into my office and said, "Dr. Madrid, they tell me these are supposed to be my golden years. I am not sure what they are talking about, but all these medicines I am on sure are costing me a lot of gold! Now I know why they call them the golden years—I am spending all of it."

Preventing chronic disease is an important step for those who are still healthy enough to do so. For those who are already struggling, simple interventions and changes can help make life healthier and more enjoyable. Unfortunately, seniors are at especially high risk for vitamin D deficiency. And those seniors who have been hospitalized are at even higher risk.

A 2005 article in the *American Family Physician* entitled, "Undiagnosed Vitamin D Deficiency in the Hospitalized Patient," discussed the prevalence of this deficiency. I could not agree more. I conduct hospital rounds on patients. Almost 100% of the patients I check have a moderate to severe vitamin D deficiency.

Mrs. Mitchell (name changed) was an 85-year old patient of mine who was hospitalized for 4 weeks due to a severe infection. She had minimal sunlight exposure during her stay, even though I would walk into her room every morning and open the blinds. Due to her overall weakness, she rarely made it outdoors to the hospital patio. I measured her vitamin D level and she was severely deficient at 8 ng/ml (20 nmol/L), a level low enough to cause rickets in children.

Mrs. Mitchell, unable to swallow medicine due to a medical problem, was receiving tube feeds. I was unable to give her vitamin D pills. I contacted the hospital pharmacy and asked if they could add 5,000 IU of vitamin D to her tube feeds. The pharmacist could not believe I was asking for such a "high dose." I explained to her that this would be OK since Mrs. Mitchell was severely deficient. I said that I personally took 5,000 IU of vitamin D daily. In spite of this, she was hesitant. We settled on adding 2,000 IU daily, and even that took some effort on my part.

A 2000 report by Dr. Michael Pfeifer (Gustav Pommer Institute in Hamburg, Germany) studied healthy elderly women over age 70 who were not hospitalized. He showed that 91% had a vitamin D level below 20 ng/ml (50 nmol/L). Today, we consider levels above 32 ng/ml (80 nmol/L) normal. Essentially, almost 100% of these senior women were deficient.

Many other studies have shown similar results. The reason for the high deficiency among senior citizens is primarily the skin's decreased ability to manufacture vitamin D, and because seniors generally tend to spend less time outdoors than younger people do. In addition, Susan Harris, DSc (Boston University School of Public Health), has demonstrated that even when senior citizens receive vitamin D supplementation, they absorb and process it more slowly than younger people.

When seniors are vitamin D deficient, they are at risk for the some of the following conditions:

- Muscle weakness
- Osteoporosis
- Falls
- Hip Fracture
- Breast cancer
- Colon cancer
- Ovarian cancer
- Heart attack
- Congestive heart failure

It is important that you have your vitamin D level checked by your family physician and start supplementing immediately. I routinely check vitamin D levels 3 months after beginning supplementation. Then, I increase or decrease the dosage until the patient reaches the desired blood level. At minimum, most seniors should be on 2,000 IU of vitamin D daily.

How to Test for Vitamin D Deficiency

Vitamin D is measured by a simple fasting or nonfasting blood test that can be done by most labs. Major labs across the country have reported increased testing for vitamin D over the last 5 years. Physicians need to order *Vitamin D-25-OH or 25-OH-D* levels. In most cases, there is no value in checking Vitamin D-1-25-OH levels, as they do not reveal a deficiency status. Minimally, levels of *vitamin D-25-OH* should be above 32 ng/ml (80 nmol/L).

Less than 10–15% of most populations have adequate levels. Levels less than 10 ng/ml (25 nmol/L) are considered severely deficient. Personally, I recommend trying to get vitamin D blood levels above 50 ng/ml (125 nmol/L) as this is where maximal cancer prevention lies, according to the studies. The upper range of normal is 100 ng/ml (250 nmol/L), although it appears that levels as high as 200 ng/ml pose no threat of toxicity. More will be discussed later about toxicity concerns.

Vitamin D Lab Values

- <10 ng/ml (<25 nmol/L) is considered severe deficiency
- 10 to 32 ng/ml (25 nmol/L-80 nmol/L) is moderate deficiency
- 33 to 49 ng/ml (82-124 nmol/L) is sufficient
- 50 ng/ml to 100 ng/ml (125 nmol/L- 250 nmol/L) is optimal for disease prevention

Sources of Vitamin D

Various foods contain vitamin D (Table 3), but not in sufficient quantity to treat a clinical vitamin D deficiency. Oily fishes such as salmon, mackerel, and sardines are good sources of vitamin D. However according to Dr. Michael Holick at a 2008 vitamin D seminar at UC San Diego, farmed fish (not in their natural habitat) may not have adequate vitamin D levels. If you eat these regularly, you can be certain that you will not get rickets. Other than that, their vitamin D levels may not be enough to prevent osteoporosis or cancer. An egg for breakfast contains about 18 IU of vitamin D, according to www.incredibleegg.org.

Cod liver oil was used to prevent rickets; however today's formulas are usually insufficient to elevate levels of vitamin D above 32 ng/ml (80 nmol/L), the lower limit of normal. Most cod liver oil supplements now provide about 20 IU of vitamin D per teaspoon, or slightly more. Today, cod liver oil is produced primarily to be a source of omega-3 fish oils.

Table 3. Vitamin D food chart.

Food	IUs per serving*	Percent DV**
Cod liver oil (traditional), 1 tablespoon	1,360	340
Salmon, cooked, 3.5 ounces	360	90
Mackerel, cooked, 3.5 ounces	345	90
Tuna fish, canned in oil, 3 ounces	200	50
Sardines, canned in oil, drained, 1.75 ounces	250	70
Milk, nonfat, reduced fat, and whole, vitamin D-fortified, 1 cup	98	25
Margarine, fortified, 1 tablespoon	60	15

Ready-to-eat cereal, fortified with 10% of the DV for vitamin D, 0.75-1 cup (more heavily fortified cereals might provide more of the DV)	40	10
Egg, 1 whole (vitamin D is found in yolk)	20	6
Liver, beef, cooked, 3.5 ounces	15	4
Cheese, Swiss, 1 ounce	12	4

(Source: National Institutes of Health. http://dietary-supplements.info.nih.gov/factsheets/vitamind.asp#h3)

Sunlight exposure is the best way to get vitamin D but requires daily exposure of face, arms, and legs between 10AM and 2PM, for 15 to 20 minutes, depending on skin pigmentation. It has been shown that between 10 AM and 2 PM, maximal UV-B light reaches the earth's surface. However, this is not always practical for most people and one's risk for skin cancer needs to be considered. The recommended daily intake (RDI) ranges from 200 IU/day up to 600 IU/day. However, because most people avoid the sun, these levels are not usually adequate to get blood levels above 32 ng/ml (80 nmol/L). In addition, studies show that these low levels of intake provide few health benefits besides rickets prevention.

Vitamin D supplementation is, therefore, very important. Depending on your blood level, you may need from 2,000 IU up to 10,000 IU daily until vitamin D deficiency disappears. Have your physician check your blood levels before beginning doses above 2,000 IU/daily.

Dosing and Toxicity of Vitamin D

Most studies have shown that 800 IU to 1,000 IU daily of vitamin D are needed for adults to see any benefit. However, blood levels are frequently deficient at these doses, so maximal benefit may not be seen. Most people need at least 2,000 IU daily of vitamin D to get their blood levels to a normal value of 32 ng/ml (80 nmol/L) or more. I personally take 5,000 IU/daily and occasionally up to 10,000 IU without problems. With this dose, I achieved a blood level of 44 ng/ml (110 nmol/L). However, have your doctor check your vitamin D blood level to ensure that the dose of vitamin D you take is sufficient. Do not just assume that since you take 2,000 IU, your body has adequate blood levels of vitamin D; it may actually be too much for you or, more likely, not enough.

One thing is certain. Most people who take 400 to 800 IU of vitamin D, the dose in multivitamins, are not getting enough vitamin D, unless they are in the sun for adequate periods of time. If you take a multivitamin, ask your doctor to check your blood level to see what it is.

A thorough review by Reinhold Vieth, PhD (University of Toronto), showed that up to 10,000 IU can be taken daily by adults without any side effects and that elevated blood calcium levels (hypercalcemia) are likely to be seen only at doses around 40,000 IU/day for extended periods. Those with lymphoma and sarcoidosis need to be careful as they are at higher risk for hypercalcemia with vitamin D supplementation.

A 2007 study in the *American Journal of Clinical Nutrition* by John N. Hathcock, PhD (Council for Responsible Nutrition), concluded: "The absence of toxicity in trials conducted in healthy adults that used a vitamin D dose > 10,000 IU supports...this value as upper intake level." The studies reviewed showed no evidence of toxicity in adults with levels as high as 10,000 IU/day of vitamin D.

In 2006, Rebecca D. Jackson, MD (The Ohio State University), and colleagues published a study in the *New England Journal of Medicine* after evaluating women enrolled in the Women's Health Initiative, a study of 36,282 women. The data showed an increased risk of kidney stones in women who took 400 IU daily in the presence of calcium when compared to women who took only calcium. How many more kidney stones? Six additional kidney stone events per 10,000 women. Other studies, however, have not corroborated this. However, even if this turns out to be true, for every 1,667 women taking vitamin D and calcium, one extra person will get a kidney stone. With numerous studies showing enormous benefits from vitamin D supplementation, this is a risk worth taking. If I ever get a kidney stone, I will be certain to post that information on my web site, vitaminD-prescription.com.

In 2007, the *New England Journal of Medicine* reported a case of a woman who had taken a product that incorrectly had too much vitamin D in it. She experienced symptoms of nausea, constipation, weakness, fatigue, and back pain. When blood levels of vitamin D were done, she was shown to be at 2,336 ng/ml (1176 nmol/L), whereas normal is 32-100 ng/ml (80 nmol/L to 250 nmol/L). The side effects she had were all related to extra calcium absorption due to the excess vitamin D.

It turned out that the manufacturer of the product had added 186,906 IU of vitamin D, or over 31,000 IU in each capsule. The patient was to take six each day. The patient was treated, did well, and was discharged after her symptoms resolved. According to the report, she died a year later from an unknown cause. However, she had a history of diabetes and rheumatoid arthritis and was, therefore, at high risk for heart disease.

This case report shows us the importance of relying on quality supplements from reputable manufacturers and the importance of checking vitamin D blood levels regularly to avoid toxicity.

Another study by John S. Adams, MD (Cedars-Sinai Medical Center and UCLA School of Medicine), reported in the *Annals of Internal Medicine* in 1997 revealed "intoxication of vitamin D." Upon further analysis, the patients were noted to have calcium in their urine and vitamin D blood levels as high as 88 ng/ml (222 nmol/L), a level now considered normal. They had no symptoms, but with extra calcium in their urine, there was a concern about the formation of kidney stones. They were instructed to discontinue the vitamin D. Upon further analysis, these patients had an increase in their bone strength, or bone density, by 1.9% per year, up to 3 years after stopping their vitamin D, illustrating the importance of vitamin D and bone strength. Stated another way, bone density increased almost 6% after 3 years.

In conclusion, vitamin D, when taken as directed, can be safe with few to no side effects. No one has ever had vitamin D toxicity from spending too much time in the sun. A person should check his or her vitamin D blood levels before beginning aggressive vitamin D supplementation. This will help to avoid toxicity and allow the person to adjust the dosage strength for maximal effectiveness. As you will see, the risks of vitamin D deficiency greatly outweigh the risks of vitamin D toxicity.

SECTION III:
RISKS OF VITAMIN D DEFICIENCY

"The best six doctors anywhere.
And no one can deny it-
Are sunshine, water, rest, and air
Exercise and diet.
These six will gladly you attend
If only you are willing
Your mind they'll ease
Your will they'll mend
And charge you not a shilling".
- Nursery rhyme quoted by Wayne Fields,
What the River Knows, 1990

Those who are deficient in vitamin D have poorer health than those who have adequate levels of vitamin D. Michael L. Melamed, MD, MHS (Albert Einstein College of Medicine, New York, USA), and colleagues conducted a study that followed over 13,000 patients for almost 9 years. The results were impressive. Those with the lowest levels of vitamin D in their blood were 26% more likely to die when compared to those with the highest levels. Do you know what your blood level of vitamin D is? Over the next several chapters, we will discuss the specific health benefits of vitamin D in additional detail.

Simply spending a little more time in the sun or supplementing your diet with vitamin D can have profound effects on your overall health. Many medical conditions respond to sunlight therapy, including seasonal affective disorder and psoriasis. The health benefits of sunshine to one's emotional well-being include triggering the brain to make hormones that improve mood, independent of vitamin D synthesis.

When I first arrived at medical school in Ohio, I had trouble getting used to the cold winters. Prior to my move to Columbus, I did not even have a winter coat. I never needed one in California; I was able to survive the "cold winters" with a sweatshirt, which surely was enough when the nighttime temperature reached a low of 50 °F (10° C).

I had to invest in a jacket, earmuffs, gloves, and a winter cap (aka beanie in Southern California). I remember thinking how much fun it would be to have a white Christmas and be able to drive in the snow. This was going to be a new experience and I was looking forward to it. The fall season was wonderful, and if this was a prelude to the winter beauty to come, I was a lucky man! Or so I thought.

By the end of November, the temperature started to fall. The nights became darker earlier and the sunshine-filled days became shorter. A little snow here or there was great. Up until this time, I had never seen snow fall. I was 25 years old and felt like a child in a candy shop.

Suddenly, without warning, winter came. I remember this cold winter as unlike no other. It was the first real winter I had experienced. I recall freezing temperatures for 6 straight weeks. The thermometer never went above 32°F (0° C). There is something inherently wrong when the inside of my freezer is warmer than outside my front door. I remember asking myself, "Why in the heck did settlers choose to stop here?" I now realized why one in 10 people in the U.S. live in California. No disrespect to people in Ohio—the birthplace of my grandparents—but the weather is for people tougher than I am.

For 6 weeks, I had to get up, go to school, study, and do my daily errands. The cold weather itself was not the worst part. However, the fact that I did not see a blue sky for 6 weeks began to wear on me. I had less energy, felt depressed, and had lost my California tan.

Finally, the day came! I saw blue sky and the daily high reached 34°F (1° C). Ice started to melt and more people around me had smiles on their faces. I literally saw a dozen people out jogging on the streets as if it were a spring day. The mood of everyone I encountered lightened up. I never thought that 34°F (1° C) would be a great day, but when one is enduring daily temperature in the teens and 20s, 34°F (1° C) becomes a godsend. It was then I started to realize the other benefits of sunshine, although I did not understand the connection with vitamin D.

Think about the last time you spent a day out in the garden soaking up the sun rays. Think about the walk you took during your lunch break instead of sitting in the artificially lighted lunchroom. How did you feel afterward? Did you feel energized? A sense of euphoria or well-being? A sense of accomplishment? Sure—just mild to moderate sunlight exposure has enormous health benefits.

The sun is the energy in the universe that gives everything life. Everyone and everything that lives and dies ultimately depends on the sun.

No fruit, vegetable, animal or person would be alive if it were not for the power of the sun. Even your dog knows how to harvest the energy from the sun as it lies out in the backyard with all four legs reaching up toward the universal light source.

We now know that those with vitamin D deficiency are at increased risk for bone demineralization, osteoporosis, muscle weakness, and muscle aches (myalgias), increased falls, fractures, chronic pain, and arthritis.

In addition, studies have shown that vitamin D deficiency during childhood increases the risk of type 1 diabetes and multiple sclerosis. Other studies have shown increased risk for heart disease, heart attacks, high blood pressure and peripheral artery disease in those who are vitamin D deficient. This information will be explored in more detail throughout the book.

Lastly, many cancers are known to be more common in those with lower vitamin D intake and lower blood levels when compared to those with higher levels.

Over the next few chapters, I will be citing studies that show the health benefits of vitamin D supplementation and increased sunlight exposure. I will also discuss a few studies that show no benefit to vitamin D supplementation, but as you will see, those studies suffered from poor design or involved insignificant doses of vitamin D.

SECTION IV:
BONE HEALTH –BONES, FALLS, FIBROMYALGIA AND CHRONIC PAIN

"I think you might dispense with half your doctors if you would only consult Dr. Sun more."
- Henry Ward Beecher 1813–1887

Bones are live organs that form the endoskeleton of vertebrates, or animals with backbones. A newborn infant has about 270 bones, many of which fuse together throughout childhood, leaving an adult with 206 fully mature bones. Bones provide strength, structure, and enable mobility. In addition, they serve as a storage site for major minerals like calcium, magnesium and phosphorus. They also store trace minerals including strontium, boron, nickel and vanadium, to name a few.

Our bones not only need these minerals for strength but also relinquish them to our blood supply so that biochemical reactions can occur. Our bones also produce important cells that are required for human life. These include red blood cells which provide energy, white blood cells to fight infections, and platelets that help our blood to clot.

When bones become thin, they are at increased risk of fracturing. When people have severely thin bones, the condition is called osteoporosis. Bone health is an important issue facing people over 50. For decades, most physicians believed that osteoporosis was a condition that primarily affected older women. However, we now know that osteoporosis also affects men, although at a lower rate. Many assume taking a calcium and vitamin D supplement in addition to routine exercise is sufficient to prevent bone disease.

While this is important, there really is more to it and, as we will see, this may not be enough to keep your bones strong.

Since the introduction of the dual energy X-ray absorptiometry (DEXA) bone density scan in the 1980s, determining one's bone density has never been easier. The DEXA scan uses a beam of X-rays that direct energy toward the bones. The result is reported as a number called a *T-Score*. With this simple bone test, people can know if they have normal healthy bones, thinning bones, or significantly porous bones (osteoporosis).

People can determine how healthy or sick their bones are and whether more action needs to be taken to strengthen their bones. Two of the more important terms you need to familiarize yourself with are osteopenia and osteoporosis.

MedicineNet.com defines osteopenia as:

> Mild thinning of the bone mass, but not as severe as osteoporosis. Osteopenia results when the formation of bone (osteoid synthesis) is not enough to offset normal bone loss (bone lysis). Osteopenia is generally considered the first step along the road to osteoporosis, a serious condition in which bone density is extremely low and bones are porous and prone to shatter.

The National Osteoporosis Foundation defines osteoporosis as:

> Osteoporosis is a disease in which bones become fragile and more likely to break. If not prevented or if left untreated, osteoporosis can progress painlessly until a bone breaks. These broken bones, also known as fractures, occur typically in the hip, spine, and wrist.

In either case, optimizing one's bone mass can provide lifelong benefits.

Risk Factors of Osteoporosis

Osteopenia and osteoporosis can affect anyone over age 40, but the older one is, the higher the risk of developing these conditions. Half of all Caucasian women will have osteopenia or osteoporosis within the first decade of menopause. Whether or not you develop these conditions is not a random event, it is something that you have control over.

Personal choices you make each and every day determine your health destiny. It is not just luck that determines who gets osteoporosis and who does not. While some may have a genetic predisposition to one disease or another, those genes need to get turned on. In most cases, genes are turned on or off by the lifestyle choices we make. Environmental factors and the lifestyle choices we make strongly determine our future health conditions.

Certain risk factors (Table 4) can increase one's risk of developing osteopenia and, ultimately, osteoporosis. Traditionally, those of Caucasian, Asian, or Hispanic heritage are at increased risk of developing this bone thinning disease. African-Americans are usually at lower risk and generally have a higher bone density when compared to Caucasians—although those of African-American heritage are still susceptible. Family history is also a risk factor. If a woman's mother has osteoporosis, that woman should take extra care to prevent developing it. While family history is a strong risk factor, it does not mean that developing osteoporosis is inevitable.

Table 4. Risk factors for osteoporosis.

Risk Factors for Osteoporosis
• Being female
• Older age
• Family history of osteoporosis
• Family history of broken bones
• Small body frame and thin build
• Certain race/ethnicities such as Caucasian, Asian, or Hispanic/Latina/o
• Personal history of broken bones at any age
• Low sex hormones - Low estrogen levels in women, including menopause, missing periods (amenorrhea) and low levels of testosterone and estrogen in men
• Diets with low calcium intake and low vitamin D intake
• Excessive intake of protein, sodium and caffeine
• Inactive lifestyle
• Smoking
• Alcohol abuse
• Certain medications such as steroid medications, seizure medicines and thyroid medicines.
• Certain diseases and conditions such as anorexia, rheumatoid arthritis and others.

(Source: National Osteoporosis Foundation http://www.nof.org/osteoporosis/disease-facts.htm)

Women who have had a hysterectomy at a young age or who are simply postmenopausal are also at risk for osteoporosis. In fact, for years, hormone replacement therapy was strongly recommended by physicians as a means to prevent osteoporosis and "maintain youth." However, a few years ago the Women's Health Initiative study came out with some alarming news that challenged the common wisdom of the day. While hormone replacement therapy with conjugated estrogens (Premarin®) helped strengthen bones and reduce fractures, it also increased the risk of breast cancer and heart attacks.

As a result, women discontinued their medications in droves and physicians became highly skeptical of writing new prescriptions for estrogen, saving them for those women who absolutely begged due to unbearable hot flashes. This example is a lesson for all. Prior to these studies, it would have been poor medicine not to prescribe the hormone replacement therapy. Today, the exact opposite is considered true.

However, the jury on hormone replacement therapy may still be out as bio-identical estrogens appear to be a safer alternative. The premise behind the bio-identical hormone replacement therapy is that the hormones are made specifically to meet the needs of the women who take them. They are compounded, or mixed, in specific concentrations as needed. They contain only one or two hormones. A big criticism of products like Premarin is that they contain numerous types of estrogens, which were extracted from **PRE**gnant **MA**re ur**IN**e, hence the name Premarin. Basically, they are hormones from horses. Is it really that surprising that women experienced negative side effects from them?

In addition to alcohol use, tobacco abuse is a huge risk factor for osteoporosis. Men and women who smoke and are over age 55 should consider having a DEXA scan. Unfortunately, most insurance companies may not cover these tests until age 65. However, if you are at risk, it may be worthwhile to get the test anyway and simply pay for it out of pocket—the cost is usually about $300.

If you smoke, stop immediately, as this can help save your bones. Ask your physician about medicines that can help you. Hypnosis and acupuncture have worked for some but are not covered by most insurance companies—in my opinion, rightfully so. If people can spend over $100 per month to smoke, they should be willing to invest at least that much to stop smoking. Smoking cessation is vital to maintaining bone health and in the prevention of osteoporosis.

I am sure you have heard the saying, *"If you don't use it, you'll lose it."* This also applies to your bones! If you are a couch potato and don't engage in moderate exercise on a regular basis (150 min/week) then your bones may be thinning out each and every single day. Lifting weights is also recommended to whatever degree possible. Even using small dumbbells to help with arm strength can be beneficial in restoring bone density and rebuilding the bone matrix.

On an Oprah Winfrey show, Dr. Mehmet Oz, of Columbia University, visited the four "Blue Zones" along with author Dan Buettner, who wrote the book *Blue Zones*. These are areas with high percentages of centenarians, or people who live past 100. In the U.S., only one city qualified—Loma Linda, California. This community is predominantly populated by Seventh-day Adventist Christians, a group where many eat a vegetarian diet. They interviewed a woman who was 104 years old and worked out with weights almost daily. This stresses the importance of weight-bearing exercises in the maintenance of bone health. When done, longevity will prevail. People over 100 in the other communities all spent adequate time in the sun producing vitamin D and were involved in daily physical activity.

Dr. Oz has done quite a bit to help promote health to the masses; he even recommends vitamin D supplementation. However, he unfortunately recommends 1,000 IU daily, a dose that most studies show is too low to significantly increase blood levels for the majority. I hope that Dr. Oz will eventually recommend that people have a vitamin D blood test to help ensure they take an adequate dose. This is really the key to optimizing vitamin D levels.

Physical inactivity, in addition to being a risk factor for premature death, is a major risk factor for osteoporosis. If you already have osteopenia or osteoporosis, talk to your doctor about beginning an exercise program to help rebuild your bone density. The health benefits of increasing physical activity are enormous and will provide you with many years of quality life.

How much will inactivity affect your bone density? Evidence shows that a person lying around in a hospital bed for as little as 1 week can lose 1-2% of his/her bone mass. For this reason, it is important that those in the hospital get physical therapy and ambulate as much as possible to help prevent the complications of lying in a hospital bed for days or weeks at a time.

Further, those who take certain medications are at increased risk for bone thinning. Some of these medications treat seizure disorders or autoimmune conditions. Many autoimmune conditions require the use of steroids such as prednisone. Steroids, when used on a regular basis can significantly increase risk for osteopenia and, ultimately, osteoporosis.

For those with autoimmune disease such as lupus erythematosus and rheumatoid arthritis, oral steroids can be lifesaving. If you have one of these conditions, it is important to keep taking your steroid medication unless your physician tells you to stop; otherwise, serious problems can occur. It is important that those who take these disease-controlling medications take extra precautions to help keep their bones strong. Eating foods high in calcium is very important. These include sesame seeds, spinach, broccoli, and almonds, to name a few. In addition, supplementing your diet with extra calcium and vitamin D is beneficial. Obtaining a DEXA bone density scan is important for those on chronic steroids. Ask your doctor if it's right for you.

A 2-year, double-blind, placebo-controlled study, reported in the *Archives of Internal Medicine* and conducted by Lenore Buckley, MD, MPH (Pediatric Rheumatologist, Richmond, Virginia), and her colleagues showed the benefits of calcium and vitamin D supplementation in those with rheumatoid arthritis. The study consisted of patients who took prednisone for their disease. The patients who took 1,000 mg of calcium carbonate and 500 IU of vitamin D daily had increased their bone density by almost 1% at the end of the study. The bones of patients who took the placebo thinned out by 0.9% to 2% per year.

Hypothyroidism is a common condition that affects about 5% (1 in 20) of the adult population. It is characterized by an underactive thyroid gland, and when present, can increase the risk of osteoporosis. If you have an underactive thyroid and are taking a thyroid replacement medicine such as levothyroxine (Synthroid®, Levoxyl®), or Armour® Thyroid, ask your doctor if a bone density scan is right for you. Also consider supplementing with additional calcium and vitamin D. **Important:** Take the calcium at least 12 hours apart from the thyroid medicine to prevent reduced absorption of your thyroid medicine.

Who Should Get a Bone Density Test?

If you have any of the risk factors listed in Table 4, ask your doctor about having a bone density test. According to the National Osteoporosis Foundation, the following people should have a bone density test:

- Postmenopausal women under age of 65 who have one or more additional risk factors, as seen in Table 4 for osteoporosis (in addition to being postmenopausal and female)
- Women age 65 and older, regardless of additional risk factors
- Postmenopausal women who sustain a fracture
- Women who are considering therapy for osteoporosis if bone density testing would facilitate the decision
- Women who have been on hormone replacement therapy (HRT/ ERT) for prolonged periods

If you have any of the above risk factors, ask your doctor for a DEXA scan, also known as a bone mineral density test. Also, have your physician check your vitamin D level.

How Osteopenia and Osteoporosis are Diagnosed

Doctors frequently diagnose osteopenia and osteoporosis when they order a routine X-ray for a patient with a suspected injury. The physician who reads an X-ray is a radiologist. Radiologists frequently report seeing either osteopenia or osteoporosis on the X-ray. The physician may recommend you get a bone density DEXA scan, as it will further classify the extent of the condition. The test will provide you with a *T-score*. The T-score (Figure 8) indicates your bone status and will let you know if you have healthy bones, osteopenia, or osteoporosis. The T-score compares your bone density to a young healthy adult of the same sex. A *Z-score* compares your bone density to others of the same age. If your T-score is between 1 and -1, then you have healthy bones. If your score is between -1 and -2.5, you have osteopenia. Scores between -2.5 and -4.5 signify osteoporosis.

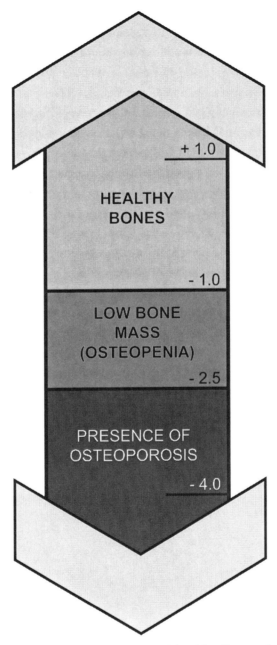

Figure 8. T scores for bone density. Healthy bones are scored from (-1 to 1), osteopenia (-1 to -2.5) while osteoporosis (-2.5 to -4.0). Illustrated by Jennifer M. Clare

Osteopenia and Osteoporosis Treatment

If a person has osteopenia, then vitamin D and calcium supplementation along with risk-factor modification should be undertaken to prevent the condition from progressing to osteoporosis. Depending on the extent of the osteopenia, your doctor may recommend a prescription medication in addition to supplements. It is important, however, to have a blood vitamin D test. If your vitamin D level is deficient, you will not appropriately absorb the calcium and bone strength will be compromised. Unfortunately, blood calcium levels do not give a good indication of calcium deficiency, so do not rely on this to determine if you need a calcium supplement.

The television is full of commercials recommending supplements and prescription medicines to help keep bones strong. From calcium supplements to pharmaceuticals drugs, the message is clear: "Reverse Bone Loss." Bisphosphonates is the main class of pharmaceutical medicines that can help reverse osteoporosis and osteopenia and rebuild bones.

Commercials recommend that patients talk to their physicians to see if Fosamax®, Actonel®, or Boniva® is right for them. However, these drugs are not without side effects. Some patients may develop an upset stomach or possibly jaw pain. Epocrates Online, a physician drug-prescribing database, lists 23 side effects possible when one takes a medicine from this class.

Side Effects of Bisphosphonates Medicines Used to Reverse Osteopenia and Treat Osteoporosis

Common Side Effects-

abdominal pain

acid reflux

nausea

dyspepsia (upset stomach)

constipation

diarrhea

musculoskeletal pain

flatulence (gas)

Serious Side Effects-

Dysphagia (difficulty swallowing)

Esophagitis (inflammation of esophagus)

Esophageal ulcer

Esophageal erosion

Esophageal perforation

Esophageal stricture

Gastric/duodenal ulcer

Hypersensitivity reaction

Angioedema (whole body swelling)

Skin reactions, severe

Hypocalcemia (low calcium)

Uveitis (eye swelling)

Scleritis (eye swelling)

Osteonecrosis, jaw (jaw bone death)

Musculoskeletal pain, severe

Source- Epocrates Drug Database (www.epocrates.com)

While these side effects appear scary, the severe reactions listed are actually quite rare. People with osteopenia or osteoporosis should ask their physicians if these medicines are appropriate for them. The majority of people who use these medicines do quite well. From my experience, an upset stomach is the biggest problem faced. In addition, it is important to weigh the risks vs. the benefits of taking these medicines. Realize that osteoporosis is a big risk factor for sustaining a hip fracture after a fall. According to the American Geriatrics Society, about 20% to 25% of those who sustain a hip fracture will die within 1 year. Some doctors may also prescribe calcitonin, a medicine that reduces bone loss.

You can see how important it is to prevent osteoporosis. If you have any of the risk factors listed in Table 4, it is important to minimize those factors to prevent premature death. Calcium supplementation is a good place to start.

Glaxo-Smith Pharmaceuticals, which produces Os-Cal®, a calcium and vitamin D supplement, cites a study on their web site that showed a 29% reduction in hip fractures when subjects took their product, which contains 400 IU of vitamin D and 1,200 mg of calcium. A 2-month supply of OsCal costs under $20.

Interestingly, Glaxo-Smith and Roche Pharmaceuticals codeveloped ibandronate (Boniva), a leading osteoporosis drug. The study cited on the Os-Cal web site did not measure vitamin D levels so we do not know whether these people were deficient. However, it is likely that most were vitamin D deficient and that the 400 IU of vitamin D did not fully correct that deficiency. Perhaps there would have been a higher reduction in hip fractures, if a stronger dose of vitamin D was given.

I have seen few drug reps promoting the inexpensive Os-Cal, but perhaps the cost of the once-monthly Boniva—$90 a pill—is partly to blame. A 3-month supply (one pill/month) of Boniva is $275 on Drugstore.com. Alendronate (Fosamax) also costs about $80 per month. In 2009, alendronate became generic, so the cost for patients should decrease.

I have never heard a drug company representative ask me if I check my patients' vitamin D levels, although low levels can lead to osteoporosis. The choice is yours; you can prevent osteoporosis for under $100/year or treat osteoporosis for $1,080/year and risk the side effects.

"But, Dr. Madrid, I have health insurance, they cover the expensive medicines. Price is not an issue. I only have a $15 co-pay." While that may be true, don't you have a premium to pay each month for your health insurance? Now you know one of the reasons your health insurance rates keep climbing year after year. Will the American health insurance industry be the next large sector needing a government bailout?

In fact, anti-osteoporosis medicine sales are big business (Table 5). In 2006, sales for osteoporosis drugs were $7 billion and they are expected to reach $10 billion by 2011. Merck alone sold $3.1 billion worth of Fosamax in 2006.

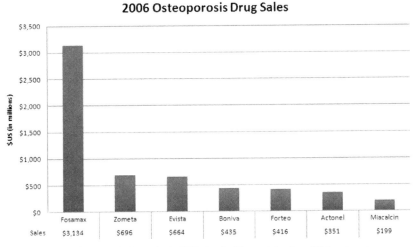

Table 5. Osteoporosis drug sales in 2006. (used with permission from WikiInvest.com)

In a patient safety brochure, Roche Pharmaceuticals, the codeveloper of Boniva, discusses the causes of osteoporosis and which type of people get osteoporosis.

EXCERPT ROCHE PATIENT SAFETY BROCHURE

Who is at risk for osteoporosis?

Talk to your health care provider about your chances for osteoporosis. Many things put people at risk for osteoporosis. The following people have a higher chance for getting osteoporosis.

Women who:

are going through or who are past menopause ("the change")

are white (Caucasian) or Asian

People who:

are thin

have a family member with osteoporosis

do not get enough calcium or Vitamin D (emphasis mine)

do not exercise

smoke

drink alcohol often

take bone-thinning medicines (like prednisone) for a long time

---

Source: http://www.rocheusa.com/products/Boniva/PI.pdf

I agree that these medicines can definitely help restore bone density and reverse osteoporosis. In addition, it is crucial that they be taken with a healthy dose of calcium and vitamin D. However, as even Roche/GSK Pharmaceuticals states, **insufficient levels of calcium and vitamin D can cause osteoporosis.**

If you already have osteoporosis, talk to your physicians about your options. These medicines in the bisphosphonate class can help improve bone strength, but it is important to check your vitamin D levels first. If they are low, you need to supplement with vitamin D to get your blood level above 32 ng/ml (80 nmol/L) and, preferably, above 50 ng/ml (125 nmol/L). Taking adequate calcium is vital; 1,200 mg/day is usually sufficient if vitamin D levels are adequate.

Can Calcium And Vitamin D Reverse Bone Loss?

Can calcium and vitamin D prevent osteoporosis and improve bone density? Certainly, it would seem that this would be too simple a solution.

According to a study in the *New England Journal of Medicine* in 1997, Bess Dawson-Hughes, MD (Former President National Osteoporosis Foundation and Professor at Tufts University School of Medicine), concluded:

> In men and women 65 years of age or older who are living in the community, dietary supplementation with calcium and vitamin D moderately reduced bone loss measured in the femoral neck, spine, and total body over the three-year study period and reduced the incidence of non vertebral fractures

A more recent study in 2004, Nicola Di Daniele, PhD (University Hospital, Tor Vergata, Rome, Italy), and colleagues in Italy concluded:

> The effect of calcium and vitamin D supplementation on bone mineral density of calcium has been demonstrated in this group of young adult women. Our results showed the positive effect of calcium and vitamin D supplementation in women both peri- and post-menopausal status; for this reason a supplementation of calcium and vitamin D should be recommended as a strategic option in helping to prevent early post-menopausal bone loss.

A study by John S. Adams, MD (Cedars-Sinai Medical Center and UCLA School of Medicine), of four patients with elevated calcium in their urine and vitamin D blood levels that averaged 88 ng/ml (220 nmol/L) found a 1.9% increase per year in bone strength (bone mineral density) over 3 years, almost 6% total. Interestingly, the patients had stopped taking their vitamin D supplements 3 years earlier after test results noted the extra calcium in their urine.

If you have not had your vitamin D level checked, what are you waiting for? Put this book down and call your physician to make an appointment. Now is the time to help build and maintain adequate bone mineral density so that you can prevent osteopenia and osteoporosis from beginning. Both men and women need to have their vitamin D levels checked. I recommend levels above 50 ng/ml (125 nmol/L) for optimal bone health.

Falls and Fractures Among Senior Citizens

When children fall, they usually get right up, shake it off, and continue playing. When young adults fall, at worst, they will usually suffer a few bruises, twist an ankle, or get a sore back. However, when a senior citizen falls, the consequences can be quite serious or even life-threatening. There are many reasons a senior citizens can fall. These include:

- Poor vision (from cataracts or macular degeneration)
- Decreased muscle strength and poor conditioning
- Light-headedness
- Carotid artery stenosis (clogged neck arteries)
- Dizziness and vertigo
- Heart disease /heart attacks
- Congestive heart failure
- Arthritis pain in knees and ankles

Whatever the cause, there is a high likelihood that elderly people will hit their heads, break bones, or cut themselves. As we age, our bones become more fragile and our skin becomes thinner. If the person happens to be on blood thinners, such as aspirin or warfarin (Coumadin®), the situation becomes more ominous. I have admitted many patients to the hospital who have passed out or tripped, only to sustain a broken hip or brain hemorrhage.

Mechanical falls from simple muscle weakness or lack of balance account for the majority of these falls. Interestingly, numerous studies have shown that low vitamin D levels are associated with increased risk of falls in senior citizens. When people supplement their diets with extra vitamin D, they can significantly reduce risks. Simple intervention can make a big difference.

As discussed, vitamin D deficiency can affect up to 90% of the elderly, especially African-American women. In addition, as people age, the skin loses the ability to produce vitamin D. A senior citizen needs to spend 3 to 5 times more time in the sun than when they were younger to produce the same amount of vitamin D. This is due to the decreased vitamin D-producing capacity of the skin and decreased absorption of ultraviolet B light (UVB). It's never too late to start supplementing your diet with vitamin D and extra calcium. If you are older than 65, vitamin D supplementation in those who are deficient can reduce the risk of falls and fractures significantly. Ask your doctor to check your vitamin D levels today.

Geriatrician Stanley J. Birge, MD (Washington School of Medicine), estimates that by the ninth decade, one in three women and one in six men will have sustained a hip fracture. These fractures are due primarily to falls in people with osteoporosis. Muscle cells have vitamin D receptors, and an adequate level of vitamin D in the blood is required for adequate muscle strength. Studies show that those who are severely deficient or simply insufficient in their vitamin D levels have decreased muscle strength and weakness, thereby providing a likely reason for excess falls.

The fall data (Table 6 below) for 2005 comes from the CDC. The right column shows the potential data I predict if physicians, insurance companies, and Medicare recommended at least biannual screening of serum vitamin D blood levels and adequate dosing of vitamin D supplementation. We can assume that upwards of 90% of the seniors who fell in 2005 were vitamin D deficient.

Table 6. Comparison of senior citizen health statistics

(A)2005 Data with 90% of Senior Citizens Vitamin D Deficient	(B) Potential Data If All Seniors Supplemented with Vitamin D for 2012
1 in 3 seniors over age 65 fell	1 in 6 seniors over age 65 fall
1.8 million ER visits due to falls	900,000 ER visits due to falls
433,000 hospitalizations due to falls	216,000 hospitalizations due to falls
16,000 seniors died from injuries sustained from the fall	8,000 seniors died from injuries sustained from a fall

Falls alone cost Medicare and private health insurance companies billions of dollars each year—not to mention the emotional costs suffered by the patients and families involved. Wouldn't the outcomes in the right column be a significant improvement?

What if your parents' lives or even your own life were saved? Would it be worth taking this "magic pill?" Of course it would! This magic pill would be considered a wonder drug and would be the number one pill taken by senior citizens. Unfortunately, this magic pill is available to all but most are not taking it. Most physicians are unaware of the benefits of this pill.

"Quality studies show that vitamin D supplementation can reduce falls and fractures from 22% to 50% in seniors"

The fact is, quality studies show that vitamin D supplementation, our magic pill, can reduce falls and fractures from *22% to 50% in seniors*. At a cost of under 10 cents/day, this would provide an enormous cost savings benefit to not only the health care system, but most importantly would increase the quality of life for millions of senior citizens and their families.

One meta-analysis (a study that reviews other studies) in a leading medical journal, *The Journal of the American Medical Association* (JAMA), involved 1,237 participants. The analysis by Heike Bischoff-Ferrari, MD, MPH (Department of Rheumatology, University Hospital Zurich), demonstrated that falls in ambulatory nursing homes or by hospitalized seniors could be reduced by at least 22% with vitamin D supplementation.

In 2003, Dr. Bischoff-Ferrari and colleagues performed a double-blind, randomized, controlled study of 122 women in a long-stay nursing home. In the study, researchers supplemented the subjects with 800 IU of vitamin D plus 1,200 mg of calcium in one group, while the control group received only 1,200 mg of calcium. The group treated with both vitamin D and calcium had a statistically significant (49%) reduced risk of falling when compared to the group who took calcium supplementation alone. The authors went on to conclude: "The impact of vitamin D on falls might be explained by the observed improvement in musculoskeletal function."

In 2003, Leon Flicker, MBBS, PhD, (University of Western Australia) and colleagues published a study of 1619 women with an average age of 84 years. The results showed senior citizens could reduce fall risk 20% when vitamin D blood levels were doubled. The researchers concluded that: "A low level of serum vitamin D is an independent predictor of incident falls."

Two years later, in 2005, Dr. Flicker (University of Western Australia) published results of their 2-year, randomized, double-blind, placebo-controlled study of 625 Australian seniors in assisted living facilities. The data, published in the *Journal of the American Geriatrics Society*, reported that those who had vitamin D levels under 36 ng/ml (90 nmol/L), but were supplemented with 1,000 IU/daily of Vitamin D, had a 27% reduction in falls. The study showed that for *each twelve people who took vitamin D, one fall each year could be prevented.*

> ## " Only eight people needed to take their vitamin D for I year to prevent one fall"

A further analysis of 540 people in the study revealed that patients who were greater than 50% compliant in taking their vitamin D showed an even greater reduction, a 37% fall risk reduction. This analysis showed that only eight people needed to take their vitamin D for 1 year to prevent one fall. Furthermore, the authors of the study concluded: "Older people in residential care can reduce their incidence of falls if they take vitamin D supplements for 2 years even if they are not initially vitamin D deficient.

The cost of vitamin D supplementation is $30 to $40 per year. Supplementing eight people with vitamin D would cost no more than $320 per year. The cost of a hip fracture, hospitalization, and repair averages $50,000 to $100,000. The cost-savings benefit is obvious. Once health insurance companies understand these numbers, vitamin D supplementation among their senior patients will, no doubt, become almost mandatory.

Lastly, a study by Dr. Michael Pfeifer (Gustav Pommer Institute in Hamburg, Germany) on the effects of vitamin D and calcium on blood levels of PTH showed that vitamin D and calcium supplementation reduced the number of falls by almost 50% after 1 year.

Not all studies show a benefit. A 2005 study in the United Kingdom included over 3,000 women at very high risk for falls. It was not a double-blind, placebo-controlled study. The study did not show any benefit in fall prevention when at-risk women received supplements of 1,000 mg of calcium and 800 IU of vitamin D. However, upon further analysis, additional flaws led many top vitamin D scientists to challenge the results. First, no one measured subjects' vitamin D blood levels. Further, the control group did not receive a placebo and, at 12 months, only 60% of the people were still taking the supplements. In addition, both participants and control group patients received handouts regarding foods high in calcium and vitamin D and provided tips for preventing falls. This intervention likely explains why both groups had fewer falls and fractures than expected, which decreased the power of the study overall.

When we evaluate well-designed studies, the evidence is clear that vitamin D supplementation and optimization of vitamin D blood levels can significantly decrease a senior citizen's risk for falling, which ultimately reduces fracture risk.

Fracture Risk Associated With Vitamin D Deficiency

Fractures are a serious and common consequence of a fall. One in four seniors who fall and break a hip will actually die within 12 months according to the American Geriatrics Society. Vitamin D supplementation not only reduces fall risk by up to 50%, it strengthens bones and reduces fractures of hips and spines.

Vitamin D is essential for calcium and phosphorus absorption in the intestines. The calcium-phosphorus complex is then able to help rebuild and strengthen the bone matrix in concert with magnesium, vitamin K, and trace minerals.

In order for bones to be healthy and strong, they must have all the main ingredients present for them to build themselves up. Much too frequently, I see patients taking over-the-counter calcium and vitamin D supplements, assuming they are getting enough. However, when we check their blood levels for vitamin D, they are deficient more often than not. I recommend ensuring a vitamin D level above 50 ng/ml (125 nmol/L) for optimal bone health. Most multivitamins and calcium/vitamin D supplements are simply inadequate to raise blood vitamin D to normal levels, that is, above 32 ng/ml (80 nmol/L).

A 2005 meta-analysis by Bischoff-Ferrari MD, MPH (Department of Rheumatology, University Hospital Zurich), in the *Journal of the American*

Medical Association showed a 26% reduction in hip fractures and a 23% reduction in any nonvertebral (nonbackbone) fractures when supplementing with 700-800 IU of vitamin D. But 400 IU of vitamin D, the dose in most vitamins, did not reduce risk.

> **"The researchers demonstrated a 37% lower risk of hip fractures in those who reportedly consumed higher levels of vitamin D"**

Diane Feskanich, ScD (Brigham and Women's Hospital and Harvard Medical School), and colleagues conducted an analysis that involved 72,337 patients. The results were published in the *American Journal of Clinical Nutrition* in 2003. The researchers demonstrated a 37% lower risk of hip fractures in those who reportedly consumed higher levels of vitamin D compared to those at lower levels. The authors of the study concluded:

An adequate vitamin D intake is associated with a lower risk of osteoporotic hip fractures in postmenopausal women. Neither milk nor a high-calcium diet appears to reduce risk. Because women commonly consume less than the recommended intake of vitamin D, supplement use or dark fish consumption may be prudent.

Significantly reduced bone loss was also seen in a double-blind, placebo-controlled study by Bess Dawson-Hughes, MD of Tufts University School of Medicine. The study evaluated 389 subjects over 65 years of age who supplemented with calcium (500 mg) and 700 IU of vitamin D. Having adequate bone density is vital to ensuring that the bones do not break during trauma. Prevention of thinning bones should begin in the 30s and 40s for both men and women.

A British randomized, double-blind placebo-controlled trial was conducted by researcher Daksha P. Trivedi and colleagues of the University of Cambridge School of Clinical Medicine. The study results showed a 22% relative risk reduction in any fracture and a 33% relative risk reduction in hip, wrist, and vertebral fractures in 2,686 men and women who were followed for 5 years. The treated subjects received 100,000 IU of vitamin D every 4 months. The results showed that 44 people needed to take a supplement to reduce any fracture, while only 29 people needed to supplement to prevent a hip, wrist, or back fracture.

In addition, this same 5-year study of seniors showed a 12% reduction in overall death in the vitamin D supplemented group—from all causes. The decreased mortality is consistent with the fact that hip fractures significantly increase risk of death within 1 year of the incident. However, that was only part of the reduction. In essence, supplementing with vitamin D decreases a senior citizen's overall risk of death by 12% over 5 years. Not a bad return for a $40-a-year investment.

With all this evidence in favor of vitamin D, surely there must be a study or two that show no benefit, right? Correct, there are. A 2006 study reported by Rebecca D. Jackson, MD (The Ohio State University), was published in the prestigious *New England Journal of Medicine*. The results showed that after 7 years of vitamin D supplementation, there was no reduction in the number of falls or fractures in postmenopausal women. However, in that study, the participants took only 400 IU of vitamin D.

A study in the *Annals of Internal Medicine,* conducted by Paul Lips, MD, PhD (University of Amsterdam), also showed no evidence of fracture prevention in seniors taking vitamin D supplementation. Dr. Lips conducted a double-blind study of 2,578 people over 70 years in age—1916 women and 662 men. The seniors were randomly assigned to receive either 400 IU of vitamin D or a placebo for up to 3 ½ years. At the end of the study, there was no difference in hip fractures.

The studies that show no benefit both used 400 IU of vitamin D. The evidence is clear; this amount is not effective. Ironically, this is close to the dose of vitamin D in most over-the-counter vitamins. Wyeth Pharmaceuticals' Centrum Silver, the leading multivitamin sold to senior citizens, actually has 500 IU of vitamin D. However, this level is still suboptimal and unlikely to affect serum levels of vitamin D to any significant degree.

It is important that all seniors have their blood levels tested for vitamin D and that supplementation with at least 2,000 IU of vitamin D be started. However, it is important to check blood levels every 3 to 6 months to maintain healthy levels, avoid toxicity, and make sure that 2,000 IU is actually enough. In my experience, most patients require 4,000 to 6,000 IU of vitamin D to get blood levels of vitamin D above 50 ng/ml (125 nmol/L).

Osteoarthritis

Osteoarthritis is a condition that occurs when the cartilage surface that coats our bones starts to deteriorate. The result is that the bone rubs against bone, bringing pain and discomfort with movement. The pain is commonly worse in the morning as the joints are stiff. As the day progresses, pain minimally improves. People frequently refer to osteoarthritis as simply *arthritis* and it commonly affects the following joints

- Knees
- Shoulders
- Hips
- Hands
- Ankles

For many senior citizens, it can limit both their daily activities and their enjoyment of life. The result is that seniors often need canes and walkers just to get around. When arthritis affects one's hand, simply opening a jar of jelly or writing a check can be a difficult task.

A patient of mine came into the office about 2 weeks before I sent my book to be published. She showed me how she was able to make a fist with her hands, without any pain. This was the first time in years she had been able to open jars and use her hands with minimal pain. Months prior, she was diagnosed with vitamin D deficiency. At the time, I was more concerned about her osteoporosis than her arthritis symptoms. However, seeing her so happy with the dexterity she had regained was rewarding.

Numerous studies show benefits of glucosamine and chondroitin sulfate, while many others have shown no benefit. My own experience with patients who use this supplement seems to be mixed; some benefit and some don't.

Nonsteroidal anti-inflammatory drugs are the main class of medicines used to treat osteoarthritis pain. Medicines in this class include ibuprofen (Motrin®, Advil®), naproxen (Aleve®), celecoxib (Celebrex®), and valecoxib (Vioxx®). Unfortunately, their high levels of side effects often limit their use. Merck's Vioxx made the headlines in 2004 when the company recalled it for causing an increased risk of heart attacks. Numerous lawsuits against Merck have followed.

> ## "Low intake and low serum levels of vitamin D appear to be associated with an increased risk for progression of osteoarthritis of the knee."

Fortunately, vitamin D can play a role in preventing osteoarthritis from developing in the first place. A study in *Annals of Internal Medicine* in 1996, conducted by Timothy McAlindon, MD (The Arthritis Center, Boston University School of Medicine) , concluded: "Low intake and low serum levels of vitamin D appear to be associated with an increased risk for progression of osteoarthritis of the knee."

A separate study by Nance E. Lan, MD (Rheumatology, University of California San Francisco), concluded low blood levels of vitamin D may be associated with x-ray changes showing hip osteoarthritis.

While there are few studies, more are sure to be underway. I am certain we will see more data over time regarding the effectiveness of vitamin D and arthritis development and the treatment of arthritis pain. In the meantime, vitamin D has numerous other benefits that should not be ignored. Overall, those with higher levels of vitamin D have less pain from any cause. Now is the time to start ensuring that your vitamin D level is adequate, as it can substantially reduce the risk of aches and pains later on in life. If you already have osteoarthritis, it would be smart to start ensuring optimal blood levels of vitamin D now, in order to prevent long-term disability and decline.

Chronic Pain and Fibromyalgia

Chronic pain and symptoms of fibromyalgia cause significant disability to hundreds of thousands of people every year. The costs associated with fibromyalgia include missed workdays and limited ability to enjoy life. Fibromyalgia, as discussed earlier, is *an increasingly recognized chronic pain ill-*

ness that is characterized by widespread musculoskeletal aches, pain, and stiffness, soft tissue tenderness, general fatigue, and sleep disturbances.

A person is diagnosed with fibromyalgia when 11 of 18 specific tender points are identified by a physician. Interestingly, the Merck Manual describes vitamin D deficiency in much the same way: Vitamin D deficiency can cause muscle aches, muscle weakness, and bone pain at any age.

There are numerous theories as to the causes of fibromyalgia, including depression and dopamine or serotonin abnormalities. Some even think the cause is an environmental toxin. In either case, it can cause many problems for the person who has it. Many are starting to think that vitamin D deficiency may play a role in fibromyalgia pain.

I have personally seen some patients with fibromyalgia symptoms improve when their vitamin D levels are optimized. However, it does not control the pain of everyone who is treated. For those people diagnosed with fibromyalgia, regular exercise has been proven effective in controlling pain. There are currently two medicines which are FDA approved for the treatment of fibromyalgia. These are pregabalin (Lyrica®) and milnacipran (Savella®). Ask your doctor what is the best treatment for you.

Adults and Chronic Pain

Millions of adults suffer from chronic pain of one type or another. Those with chronic nonspecific pain syndromes, osteomalacia (soft bones), and fibromyalgia can benefit from vitamin D supplementation. Several studies have shown an increased risk of myalgias and generalized body pains in those deficient in vitamin D.

According to a case report by Anu Prabhala, MD (Division of Endocrinology, Diabetes, and Metabolism, State University of New York at Buffalo), vitamin D therapy improved the lives of five people with severe disabilities and difficulty walking. Two were elderly and had severe muscle weakness, requiring a wheelchair just to get around. Once the vitamin deficiencies were identified and appropriate vitamin D treatments administered, the pain and weakness resolved in four of the five people over 4 to 6 weeks. The four then became fully mobile, while the fifth became partially mobile.

> ## "People who were vitamin D deficient needed almost two times more pain medicine to control their pain."

A study reported by Sherry Boschert in *Family Practice News*, 2008, showed that those patients with chronic pain and lower vitamin D blood levels required higher doses of pain medicine to control their pain and have been using pain medicines for a longer period of time when compared to patients with higher levels of vitamin D. "People who were vitamin D deficient needed almost two times more pain medicine to control their pain."

In fact, those who were deficient in vitamin D required an average of 134 mg/day of morphine equivalents compared with 70 mg/day of morphine equivalents in those who had higher blood levels of vitamin D, almost two times more. It is interesting to note that this study defined a normal vitamin D level as being greater than 20 ng/ml (50 nmol/L), while most physicians and labs use 32 ng/ml (80 nmol/L) as the cutoff level. In other words, the effects could have been even more dramatic had they referred to the higher blood level in the study.

Research by Greg Plotnikoff, MD, FACP (Clinical Medicine and Pediatrics, University of Minnesota Medical School), studied 150 patients with chronic, nonspecific musculoskeltal pain. All patients were nonresponsive to traditional therapy. Dr. Plotnikoff found that 93% of patients were vitamin D deficient with levels less than 20 ng/ml (50 nmol/L). He recommended that since "osteomalacia is a known cause of persistent, nonspecific musculoskeletal pain, screening all outpatients with such pain for hypovitaminosis D should be standard practice in clinical care."

A 2003 study conducted in Saudi Arabia, by Al Faraj, MD and published in the *Journal of Spine*, showed that 93% of 341 patients with chronic lower back pain with no specific cause improved after vitamin D supplementation; and 83% (299 patients) of those with the pain were clinically deficient at the start. Women in Arab countries are at high risk for vitamin D deficiency because they cover themselves for religious reasons with burqas. The authors of the study concluded:

> Vitamin D deficiency is a major contributor to chronic low back pain in areas where vitamin D deficiency is endemic. Screening

for vitamin D deficiency and treatment with supplements should be mandatory in this setting. Measurement of serum (Vitamin D) 25-OH cholecalciferol is sensitive and specific for detection of vitamin D deficiency, and hence for presumed osteomalacia in patients with chronic low back pain.

One small study by Robert Sweezy, MD (Arthritis and Back Pain Center, Santa Monica, California), compared 23 women with fibromyalgia to 46 women of similar age, without fibromyalgia. The authors concluded:

> Fibromyalgia in this…study was frequently associated with osteoporosis. Early detection and implementation of appropriate nutritional supplementation (calcium/vitamin D), resistive and weight bearing exercise, and specific bone mineral enhancing pharmacological therapy can be indicated in pre, peri, and postmenopausal subjects.

Although the study did not measure the vitamin D levels in these patients, it is very likely that those with fibromyalgia had lower levels than the controls based on my personal experience with my fibromyalgia patients.

Growing Pains in Children

Growing pains are a common complaint of children all across the world. What if growing pains were simply the result of a vitamin D deficiency? This might not be too far from the truth.

A study reported by Jane Salodof MacNeil and published in *Family Practice News* described 41 children with nonspecific musculoskeletal pain. The vitamin D blood levels were significantly lower in 35 of the children with vague pain (~28 ng/ml) than in the remaining 6 children (38 ng/ml), whose cause of pain was determined. Furthermore, when eight of the children took vitamin D supplements, five experienced significant improvement or complete loss of pain. In fact, the study showed that 30% of the children, all living in New Mexico, had vitamin D blood levels below 25 ng/ml (62.5

nmol/L). We used to assume that those in the sunshine states got enough sun, but this study clearly shows otherwise.

We need to see more studies in these fields before we can make definite conclusions about fibromyalgia or growing pains in children. However, the above studies do introduce some interesting possibilities about future therapies for chronic pain. If you suffer from chronic pain, ask your physician to measure your vitamin D blood level.

SECTION V:
INFECTIONS, YOUR HEART, AND HORMONES

"To wish to be well is a part of becoming well."
- (Roman philosopher, mid-1st century AD)

Influenza and Tuberculosis

Head colds, influenza infections, and tuberculosis affect millions of people annually worldwide. Cold and flu viruses commonly infect more people during the winter season. For this reason, many healthcare professionals recommend that those at risk, such as senior citizens and diabetics, take their flu shots annually. As a matter of fact, this is the recommendation of most professional medical associations, including the American Medical Association. Patients flock to their doctors and pharmacies starting in early November asking for the "lifesaving vaccine." They continue to ask up until about late February.

Our parents and grandparents told us, "Make sure you put on your jacket before you go out or you're going to catch a cold." Does cold weather really make people sick? I thought it was only viruses and bacteria that make people sick. At least that is what I learned in medical school. What does cold weather have to do with catching a cold? Many assume that this is an old wive's tale.

For years, the "intelligent" countered this tale with the assumption that upper respiratory viruses are passed along more during the cold months because people stay indoors more, allowing more intimate contact, and therefore sharing germs. Whether or not one wore a jacket was irrelevant.

> ## "Vitamin D supplementation could prevent one from developing the flu"

In 1965, Dr. Edgar Hope-Simpson (1908-2003), a general practitioner, was given credit for proposing that the shingles infection was caused by reactivation of the chicken pox virus. In 1981, he proposed that solar radiation (sunshine) could protect against the flu virus. In 2006, Dr. John Cannell (Vitamin D expert and psychiatrist at Atascadero State Hospital, California) and colleagues published a paper showing evidence that lower vitamin D blood levels during the winter can account for the increased transmissibility of the influenza virus among children and adults. This, along with numerous other studies about vitamin D, started a paradigm shift.

Studies show that vitamin D stimulates the immune system and disease-fighting cells, called macrophages and T cells. The cells create proteins that have antiviral and antimicrobial properties. Further, we know that macrophages and T cells have vitamin D receptors (VDRs) on them, enhancing their functions. Dr. Cannell became interested in vitamin D research when he noted that patients in his psychiatric ward who took 2,000 IU of vitamin D did not get the flu, while the patients in other wards (who did not take vitamin D) did. The patients intermingled with each other so cross exposure was certain. The study showed that vitamin D supplementation could prevent one from developing the flu.

Tuberculosis, a disease "of old," is unfortunately reappearing in the U.S. and Europe. Fortunately, adequate health care and access to antituberculosis drugs make controlling this disease easier than in times past. However, the TB bacteria infects up to 40% of the world's population who simply don't have access to the medicines found in industrialized countries. The poor sanitary conditions and crowded living quarters commonly seen in most third-world countries aid in the contagiousness and transmissibility of TB. Interestingly, studies have shown that vitamin D, when taken with appropriate antituberculosis medications, can help achieve higher TB cure rates than with antibiotics alone. A study reported by Alvin Powell in the *Harvard Gazette* cited research that showed that those of African descent are more susceptible to TB, due to lower vitamin D blood levels, and that vitamin

D supplementation, thru enhancing the immune system, can suppress TB infection from occurring.

Further, a study in *The Lancet* of children in Ethiopia evaluated 500 children under the age of 5 with pneumonia. Of these, 210 also had rickets due to low vitamin D and calcium intake. Researchers compared these children to 500 children admitted for something other than pneumonia. The researchers concluded that those with rickets were 13 times more likely to develop pneumonia. These findings indicate a connection between vitamin D status, immune system, and infection susceptibility.

While there is still a lot of research to do in this field, the implications are enormous. If more studies support the antibacterial and antiviral effects of vitamin D, the benefits to human health will prove to be priceless. Human morbidity and mortality can be diminished at a cost of pennies per day. Ensuring adequate vitamin D supplementation during the winter may help prevent the next flu epidemic or pneumonia from killing millions of people worldwide. Further, those who are at risk for TB can be treated for only pennies per day.

Hyperparathyroidism

The parathyroid, which consists of four small glands, sits on the back of the thyroid gland in the neck, below the Adam's apple. The purpose of the parathyroid is to regulate the blood's calcium levels. When the parathyroid generates too much of its hormone, parathyroid hormone (PTH), the condition is called hyperparathyroidism. This is usually the result of either a benign (noncancerous) growth of the thyroid gland or from vitamin D deficiency.

Hyper = more than normal

parathyroid = gland

ism = condition

When our bodies are deficient in vitamin D, the gut is unable to absorb calcium in sufficient amounts. In response, our bodies produce excess PTH, which releases calcium from our bones. This phenomenon is called secondary hyperparathyroidism. This helps ensure that our blood level of calcium will remain stable, allowing muscles to contract and biochemical reactions to occur. For this reason, a blood test is not a good indicator of calcium insufficiency. This explains why many men and women with osteoporosis have normal calcium on blood tests.

A study by Dr. Michael Pfeifer (Gustav Pommer Institute in Hamburg, Germany) on the effects of vitamin D and calcium on blood levels of PTH shows that vitamin D and calcium supplementation help bring levels of PTH closer to normal.

If a person's PTH does not correct after replenishing vitamin D, it is important that a doctor evaluate the patient for a benign parathyroid tumor or, rarely, a cancerous tumor. When a tumor makes extra PTH, the condition is called primary hyperparathyroidism.

Kidney Disease

Most people have two kidneys, one on each side. The kidneys help control fluid balance; filter blood; regulate electrolytes, such and sodium and potassium; and help remove toxins, including urea, from the blood. Urea, a product of protein breakdown, is where we get the word urine. The kidneys drain liquid waste into the bladder though the ureters, the tubes that connect the kidneys to the bladder. The waste products are then expelled when one urinates. Kidneys are also instrumental in controlling blood pressure, producing hormones that make red blood cells, and activating vitamin D.

Kidneys can be healthy or diseased. A healthy kidney filters blood at a rate of 90 ml/min or more. Diseased kidneys filter less than this or they may abnormally excrete protein, which can be measured in the urine. High blood pressure and diabetes are major risk factors for kidney disease. The National Kidney foundation estimates that 26 million Americans have kidney disease and millions of other people are at risk for developing kidney disease. The US Renal Data System estimated that in 2006, 110,851 new cases of End Stage Renal Disease (ESRD) were diagnosed. There are five stages of kidney disease, each stage depends on the amount of blood a kidney is able to filter per minute. Stage 1 kidney disease is the mildest form, while Stage 5, ESRD, is the most serious.

- Stage 1- kidney filters blood greater than 90 ml/min but there is protein in the urine.
- State 2- mild, kidney filters blood at a rate of 60 to 89 ml/min

- Stage 3- moderate, kidney filters blood at a rate of 30-59 ml/minute
- Stage 4- severe, filters blood at a rate of 15-29 ml/minute
- Stage 5- very severe, ESRD, kidney filters blood at a rate of less than 15 ml/min. May need dialysis due to kidney failure

When people experience Stage 5 kidney disease, the situation becomes grave. They often need to be on kidney dialysis just to survive. People on kidney dialysis are connected to a machine, three times a week, that filters their blood. This removes toxins that a healthy kidney would normally remove.

The data shows that 10% to 40% of people with diabetes and high blood pressure will develop kidney disease between Stages 1 through 5. According to NIH, in the U.S. alone, 50 million people have hypertension; there are 1 billion afflicted worldwide. The U.S. Renal Data System reports that every year, high blood pressure causes 25,000 cases of kidney failure. This is why reversing your diabetes and controlling blood pressure are very important.

Those with chronic kidney disease are frequently vitamin D deficient. The primary reason is that the kidney contains an enzyme that converts vitamin D-25OH to vitamin D 1,25 OH. A diseased kidney is unable to do this effectively. There is no evidence that vitamin D deficiency causes kidney disease, but those with kidney disease have a high likelihood of having vitamin D deficiency.

There is evidence that vitamin D supplementation can help those with kidney disease. A study conducted by Nephrologist, Dr. Ming Teng (Fresenius Medical Care North America, Lexington) and his colleagues appeared in the *Journal of the American Society of Nephrology*. The study showed that patients receiving renal dialysis (Stage 5 disease) and vitamin D replacement had lower death rates overall than those who did not receive the vitamin D replacement. In addition, they were half as likely to have a stroke or heart attack. This led the authors to conclude, "In this historical cohort study, chronic...dialysis patients in the group that received...vitamin D had a significant survival advantage over the patients who did not."

If you have kidney disease of any sort, ask your family physician or kidney specialist, to check your vitamin D level and whether vitamin D supplementation is right for you. Those with more advanced kidney disease may need a vitamin D analogue prescribed to them instead of the usual over the counter vitamin D supplement.

Important: Those on dialysis or with advanced renal disease should work closely with their physicians, as they are at higher risk for electrolyte abnormalities. If you have kidney disease, you should take vitamin D supplementation only under the guidance of your physician.

Cardiovascular Disease Risk

Cardiovascular disease comprises any disease that affects the heart and arteries. Those who have it are at risk for strokes, heart attacks, congestive heart failure, and peripheral vascular disease. Major risk factors of cardiovascular diseases include *high blood pressure, diabetes, obesity*, smoking, family history, high cholesterol, and lack of physical activity. Of these, the first three are also associated with vitamin D deficiency.

High Blood Pressure

The terms *high blood pressure* and *hypertension* refer to the same thing. Hypertension is a condition in which the heart has to pump harder than usual due to increased pressure and stiffness in arteries. This condition affects about 50 million Americans, or 1 in 4 adults.

Hypertension, considered a "silent killer" by many health professionals, is a leading risk factor for heart disease and cardiac death. Hypertension affects 50 million Americans and 1 billion people worldwide. There are few or no symptoms associated with hypertension, yet having it puts one at higher risk for dying from the top killing diseases. There are two main types of hypertension. *Essential hypertension* accounts for 90% of all hypertension and has no one specific cause. *Secondary hypertension*, whose cause can be determined by a doctor, accounts for the remaining 10%.

Hypertension is known to increase the risk of heart attacks and congestive heart failure (No. 1 killers in the U.S.), stroke (No. 3 killer in the US) and kidney disease (No. 9 killer in the U.S.), especially if left untreated. The dangers of hypertension and its effects are seen all over the world.

Your blood pressure consists of two numbers, traditionally measured in millimeters of mercury. The first number is the systolic (pronounced si-**stol**-ik) pressure and the second number is the diastolic (pronounced die-uh-**stol-**ik) pressure. Blood pressure appears as 120/80 (120 over 80). The bigger number is the systolic blood pressure and the smaller number is the diastolic, always. The systolic pressure is the pressure your heart exerts on your arteries when pumping, whereas the diastolic is the pressure in the arteries when your heart relaxes.

> **Normal Blood Pressure**
> <u>120</u> = systolic
> 80 = diastolic

To determine if you have hypertension, you should have your family physician check it. To make the diagnosis, a person must have two readings at rest, while sitting with both feet on the ground. The measurements should be taken at least 5 minutes apart. Two values greater than 140/90 indicate hypertension. If you check your blood pressure at home with a digital blood pressure cuff or at a local drugstore and your numbers exceed 140/90, call your doctor immediately.

> **High Blood Pressure**
> <u>140</u> = systolic
> 90 = diastolic

When the blood pressure is high, the heart has to work harder to pump blood throughout the body. Since the heart is a muscle, if it works harder it will get bigger. Although most of us usually want bigger muscles, having a bigger heart is not a good idea. When the heart becomes enlarged, a person runs the risk of developing heart arrhythmias (irregular heartbeats), congestive heart failure, or other heart problems.

Evidence shows that, by lowering blood pressure to 120/80, people can significantly reduce the risk of heart attack and stroke. When this is accomplished, people will live longer and enjoy a higher quality of life. If you have high blood pressure, this should be your goal.

There are many factors that can contribute to high blood pressure. These include stress, poor diet, overweight, obesity, diabetes, alcohol abuse, magnesium deficiency, lack of exercise, family history, and old age. Kidney disease and hormone imbalances can also raise blood pressure. By correcting these risk factors, people can significantly improve blood pressure.

A discussion about these factors is beyond the scope of this book. Interestingly, vitamin D deficiency is also associated with hypertension. Optimizing our internal environment is crucial to obtaining overall health.

Risk factors for high blood pressure:

- Stress
- Poor diet
- Vitamin D deficiency
- Overweight
- Obesity
- Diabetes
- Alcohol abuse
- Magnesium deficiency
- Lack of exercise
- Family history
- Old age
- Kidney disease
- Adrenal gland tumors

Studies show that those with lower levels of vitamin D are at higher risk for hypertension. Several studies have shown that those with lower vitamin D blood levels have higher blood renin levels, a chemical that raises blood pressure. While controlling and identifying all the other causes is important, treating a vitamin D deficiency is crucial in bringing balance back to our bodies.

A report by Mitchell Zoler, in *Family Practice News* quoted Dr. John P. Forman at the 2006 annual meeting for the American Society for Hypertension as saying, "We conclude that serum levels of 25-hydroxyvitamin D (vitamin D) may be an independent risk factor for incident hypertension."

Dr. Forman and colleagues published a report in the *Journal of Hypertension* about two studies, one that lasted 4 years and one that lasted 8 years. They compared men and women who had vitamin D blood levels below 15 ng/ml (37.5 nmol/L) vs. those with blood levels above 30 ng/ml (75 nmol/L). The results were clear. *Men with lower levels of vitamin D were 6 times more likely to have hypertension.*

> ## "Men with lower levels of vitamin D were 6 times more likely to have hypertension while woman were almost 3 times more likely to have hypertension"

When researchers looked at the women, they found that women with vitamin D levels below 15 ng/ml were almost 3 times more likely to have hypertension compared to those with normal levels of vitamin D.

The researchers were careful to make sure they factored in age, activity level, weight, and BMI to make sure the results were accurate, and they did not change. The message is clear; higher vitamin D levels in the blood can prevent high blood pressure.

The questions then becomes, how does vitamin D lower blood pressure? What is the mechanism of action?

Yan Chun Li, PhD (University of Chicago) showed in his study that vitamin D actually turns off the genes (acting via VDRs, the vitamin D receptors) that create the chemical renin, which raises blood pressure. It is interesting to note that the author of the study went on to conclude that vitamin D analogues (look-alike molecules) could help treat high blood pressure. Basically, if vitamin D can help lower blood pressure, why should we rely on expensive, patented, look-alike molecules to lower blood pressure? Vitamin D treatments for blood pressure control will likely become a new area for scientific research.

What is my recommendation? If you have hypertension, make sure you work hard to control it. Your physician may prescribe blood pressure medicines, which act to lower the amount of work your heart needs to do. Common blood pressure medications prescribed to help control blood pressure include:

- Diuretics such as hydrochlorothiazide, triamterene and aldactone work to remove excess sodium from the blood and therefore lower blood pressure
- Beta blockers such atenolol, metoprolol (Toprol®), carvedilol (Coreg®) work on the heart and blood vessels to lower blood pressure
- Calcium channel blockers such as amlodipine (Norvasc®), nifedipine (Procardia®) cause blood vessels to open, resulting in lower blood pressure
- Ace inhibitors such as lisinopril and benazapril work to lower the artery resistance and block a chemical called renin, which raises blood pressure
- Angiotensin Receptor Blockers such as losartan (Cozaar®) and olmesartan (Benicar®) block a chemical, allowing the blood vessels to widen

You should never stop taking your blood pressure medicine unless instructed to do so by your health care provider. Vitamin D does not interact with any of the above blood pressure medicines.

Second, ask your doctor to check your vitamin D level. If appropriate, take at least 2,000 IU daily of vitamin D and recheck your blood level after 3 months. Third, eat a diet high in fruits and vegetables. Foods high in magnesium such as black beans, spinach, and pumpkins seeds can also help lower blood pressure. In addition, regular exercise, meditation, and maintaining a healthy weight will do a lot for you in your quest to control your blood pressure.

> **"Foods high in magnesium such as black beans, spinach, and pumpkins seeds can also help lower blood pressure"**

Remember, regular doctor visits are extremely important to make sure your blood pressure is well controlled. A holistic approach using diet, exercise, medicines and supplements can go a long way in helping you control your blood pressure.

Heart Disease

Heart disease, an inflammatory disease of the heart and arteries, is the leading killer in the U.S. Having high blood pressure is a leading risk factor. As a matter of fact, over 900,000 Americans die from complications related to heart disease each year, including sudden cardiac death from heart attacks and congestive heart failure, a condition that occurs when the heart stops pumping blood adequately to the body. To break it down into simpler terms, 100 people each hour die in the U.S. from heart disease and related conditions. What if we could reverse this trend?

Worldwide, about 46,000 people die each day from heart attacks. This equates to 1,916 people each hour, or 30 people each minute. Controlling risk factors are vital in the prevention of heart attacks.

Risk factors for heart disease, in no particular order, include the following:

- Lack of exercise
- Family history
- Obesity
- High blood pressure
- Tobacco use
- High cholesterol
- Elevated cardiac CRP
- Elevated homocysteine
- High fat diet
- Diabetes
- Vitamin D deficiency

Only recently has vitamin D deficiency been added to the list of heart attack risk factors. A primary reason for this was due to research by Thomas J. Wang, MD (Department of Medicine, Massachusetts General Hospital, Harvard Medical School) and colleagues. They published a study in

Circulation in 2008 that showed people with lower levels of vitamin D in their blood were at higher risk for heart attacks when compared to people with higher vitamin D levels. In his study, he concluded, "Vitamin D deficiency is associated with incident cardiovascular disease."

> **"Those with vitamin D levels below 10 ng/ml (25 nmol/L) had an 80% increased risk of heart attack when compared to those with vitamin D levels above 15 ng/ml"**

Dr. Wang showed that those with a vitamin D level between 10 ng/ml (25 nmol/L) and 15 ng/ml (37.5 nmol/L) had a 53% increased risk of heart attack when compared to those with vitamin D levels above 15 ng/ml (37.5 nmol/L). Those with vitamin D levels below 10 ng/ml (25 nmol/L) had an 80% increased risk of heart attack when compared to those with vitamin D levels above 15 ng/ml.

In 2008, Edward Giovannucci, MD, ScD (Harvard School of Public Health), published in the *Archives of Internal Medicine* a study which showed that people with vitamin D levels less than 15 ng/ml (37.5 nmol/L) were over 2 times more likely to have a heart attack when compared to those with vitamin D levels above 30 ng/ml (75 nmol/L).

Further, a German study published in 2008 by Dr. Stefan Pilz and colleagues (Department of Public Health, Social and Preventive Medicine, Mannheim Medical Faculty, University of Heidelberg) showed even more astonishing results. From 1997 to 2000, Dr. Pilz measured vitamin D blood levels in 3,299 men with heart disease—men whose doctors recommended heart catheterizations or angiograms to evaluate the severity of their disease. After following these patients for almost 8 years, it was shown that those with vitamin D levels less than 10 ng/ml (25 nmol/L) were almost 3 times more likely to die from heart failure when compared to those with vitamin D blood levels above 30 ng/ml (75 nmol/L). Furthermore, those with lower vitamin D blood levels were 5 times more likely to die from sudden cardiac death when compared to those with higher levels. The authors went on to conclude:

Low levels of vitamin D are associated with prevalent myocardial dysfunction (heart disease), deaths due to heart failure and sudden cardiac death. Interventional trials are warranted to elucidate whether vitamin D supplementation is useful for treatment and/or prevention of heart diseases.

Basically, they concluded that low levels will kill you, but that more studies are needed to see whether treatment will save your life. As I see it, you have two choices if you suffer from heart disease. First, you can check your vitamin D levels and then supplement to make sure your blood levels are optimized or, second, you can wait 2 to 10 years (if you are still around) and see what future studies show. The choice is obvious. Ask your doctor to check your vitamin D level. Supplementation with at least 2,000 IU of vitamin D is strongly encouraged.

It is also important to minimize the other listed risk factors. It is only when all these risk factors are addressed, significant health improvement can occur. Stop smoking, eat more fruits and vegetables, consume a low inflammatory diet, lose weight, and become more physically active. By doing so, you will add quality years to your life.

Peripheral Artery Disease

Another indicator of severe heart disease is peripheral artery disease. This is diagnosed in people who develop bad pain in their legs with mild exercise, or simply walking; and is the result of poor blood flow due to clogged leg arteries. When this occurs, one can be almost certain that the arteries of the heart also have blockage.

A study by Michael L. Melamed, MD, MHS (Albert Einstein College of Medicine, New York, USA), and colleagues published in *Arteriosclerosis, Thrombosis, and Vascular Biology* in 2008 concluded that "low serum vitamin D is associated with a higher prevalence of peripheral artery disease." In fact, the study showed that those with the lowest levels were 80% more likely to have poor blood circulation when compared to those with the highest levels.

While this is only one study on peripheral artery disease and vitamin D, this study is consistent with other studies on cardiovascular disease. It is important, however, to make sure you get your vitamin D levels checked; don't assume that since you are taking a multivitamin, or even a vitamin D supplement, that you are getting enough.

Some Studies Show No Benefit

A study by Judith Hsia, MD (George Washington University) and colleagues of 36,282 women who took 400 IU daily of vitamin D showed no benefit in preventing heart disease or strokes with vitamin D. This result is not surprising. As with other study results, we know that 400 IU of vitamin D will not significantly alter one's blood level. Curiously, this is the level of vitamin D found in most leading over-the-counter supplements.

This area of vitamin D research and heart disease is a growing field. It is likely that scientists will be publishing more studies in the years to come, especially as people are trying to focus more on the prevention of cardiovascular disease.

OBESITY

Obesity is a leading risk factor for cardiovascular disease and diabetes. It is a condition that affects almost one third of the adult population, while an additional one-third is overweight. Today, only one in three people is considered normal weight. A person with a BMI greater than 30 is considered obese. Obesity is a major risk factor associated with diabetes and numerous other health issues, including heart attacks and cancer. Being overweight severely affects one's quality of life. Experts believe that, because of obesity, the generation of children born today will actually have a shorter lifespan than their parents.

> **"The generation of children born today will actually have a shorter lifespan than their parents"**

Are you considered normal weight, overweight, or obese? Most people who are obese actually believe that they are not. I recommend you calculate your BMI using the chart (Figure 9).

On the left side of the chart, find your height; on the top, find your weight. Find your number between 13 and 60. This is your BMI.

Height in Feet and Inches	Weight In Pounds													
	120	130	140	150	160	170	180	190	200	210	220	230	240	250
4'6"	29	31	34	36	39	41	43	46	48	51	53	56	58	60
4'8"	27	29	31	34	36	38	40	43	45	47	49	52	54	56
4'10"	25	27	29	31	34	36	38	40	42	44	46	48	50	52
5'0"	23	25	27	29	31	33	35	37	39	41	43	45	47	49
5'2"	22	24	26	27	29	31	33	35	37	38	40	42	44	46
5'4"	21	22	24	26	28	29	31	33	34	36	38	40	41	43
5'6"	19	21	23	24	26	27	29	31	32	34	36	37	39	40
5'8"	18	20	21	23	24	26	27	29	30	32	34	35	37	38
5'10"	17	19	20	22	23	24	26	27	29	30	32	33	35	36
6'0"	16	18	19	20	22	23	24	26	27	28	30	31	33	34
6'2"	15	17	18	19	21	22	23	24	26	27	28	30	31	32
6'4"	15	16	17	18	20	21	22	23	24	26	27	28	29	30
6'6"	14	15	16	17	19	20	21	22	23	24	25	27	28	29
6'8"	13	14	15	17	18	19	20	21	22	23	24	25	26	28
	Healthy Weight				Overweight					Obese				

Figure 9. Body Mass Index (BMI) chart.
Compiled by Jonathan Madrid

Write your BMI here: _____

BMI Interpretation:

- <18.5 is considered underweight
- 18.5 to 25 is normal healthy weight
- 25.1 to 30 is overweight
- 30.1 to 40 is obese
- 40.1 or more is considered morbidly obese

Obesity is a known risk factor for being deficient in vitamin D. In fact, perhaps as much as 80% of all obese people are vitamin D deficient, according to a study by Elina Hyppönem, PhD, Centre for Paediatric Epidemiology and Biostatistics, Institute of Child Health, London.

Since vitamin D is a fat-soluble vitamin, it appears that those with more fat store more vitamin D in their fat cells. The result, their blood levels are low. This fact has led Dr. Michael Holick of Boston University to state that fat acts like a "sink" for vitamin D. In my own medical practice, about 90% of my patients who are obese lack adequate vitamin D in their blood.

In a 2000 study by Jacobo Wortsman, MD (Southern Illinois University School of Medicine), published in the *American Journal of Clinical Nutrition,* it was shown that obese people had 57% lower vitamin D blood levels compared to non-obese people. Dr. Wortsman concluded that vitamin D was lower in obese people because it was deposited in fat tissue throughout the body.

Whatever your weight is, it is important to check your blood level of vitamin D, and if not optimal, then increase sunlight exposure and start your vitamin D supplements today. Increasing vitamin D blood levels will help reduce, in part, the risk that being overweight and obesity plays for certain diseases, especially diabetes. Also, if you are considered overweight or obese, talk to your physician about starting a weight loss program and seeing a certified nutritionist.

Diabetes Mellitus – An Overview

There are two main types of diabetes mellitus, type 1 diabetes and type 2 diabetes. Diabetes is epidemic worldwide, affecting over 150 million individuals and their families.

Type 1 diabetes—traditionally referred to as *juvenile onset*—accounts for 5% to 10% of all diabetes cases. In this type of diabetes, an autoimmune reaction affects the pancreas. The pancreas is unable to produce the insulin that helps sugar get into muscles and other cells of the body. This results in elevated blood sugars levels, or diabetes. Consequently, an affected person must begin insulin injections immediately; otherwise, they can become seriously ill or even die.

This often confuses families, as the children are usually thin and eat relatively healthy foods. Unfortunately, there is little to do to reverse this type of diabetes once it occurs. However, prevention of type 1 diabetes may be possible. I will discuss more about this later.

Type 2 diabetes—generally referred to as *adult onset* diabetes—accounts for 90-95% of all cases of diabetes. People who develop type 2 diabetes usually do so because of poor lifestyle choices. They are usually able to control their blood sugar with pills and diet. However, in some, even this fails and they must take insulin. Type 2 diabetes is commonly seen in people who have poor eating habits and fail to exercise regularly. For most, lifestyle changes, diet restriction, and a little motivation can help reverse this type of diabetes. I have seen it happen many times.

Those who do not control their diabetes, significantly increase their risk for heart attacks, strokes, blindness, kidney disease, peripheral artery disease, nerve damage, amputation, and premature death. Those with poorly controlled diabetes can expect to die up to 10 years earlier than they would if they did not have the disease.

The unfortunate thing, however, is that most of us physicians fail to inform our patients that they can reverse this type of diabetes. Patients often assume they will be relying on medicines for the rest of their lives. I am often amazed when I tell patients we can cure their diabetes. They look at me like I've just given them the "Secret of Life." While I frequently use the term "cure," other doctors prefer to consider these patients as having "diet-controlled diabetes." It is a matter of semantics. Whatever word is used, the person essentially eliminates the disease state from their body, but must be careful to ensure it does not return, as they are always very susceptible.

A study by David J. Di Cesar, MD (State University of New York, Upstate Medical University, Syracuse), showed 63.5% of Type 2 diabetics were vitamin D deficient; whereas 36% of type 1 diabetics were vitamin D deficient. The actual numbers are higher since, in his study, levels under 20 ng/ml (50 nmol/L) were considered deficient, while most labs today use 32 ng/ml (80 nmol/L) as normal.

Percentage of Diabetes Patients with Vitamin D Deficiency

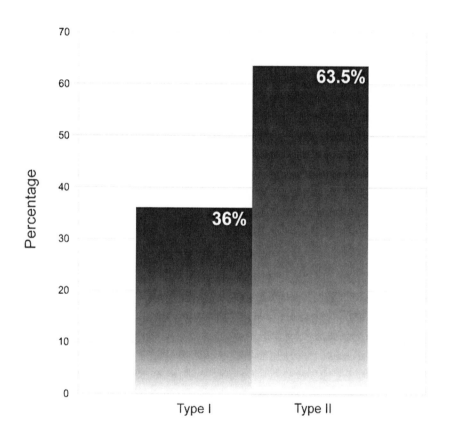

Table 7. Vitamin D Deficiency common in over 63.5% of Type II diabetes and at least 36% of Type I diabetics. Illustrated by Jennifer M. Clare

These statistics should be of concern, not only to every physician who treats diabetic patients, but even more importantly, to everyone who has diabetes. Even using the low level of 20 ng /ml as normal, 2 out of 3 patients with type 2 diabetes were deficient in vitamin D as were about 1 in 3 type 1 diabetics. If you, or a family member, have diabetes, call your doctor for a vitamin D blood test today.

Type 1 Diabetes Mellitus

The less frequent juvenile onset (type 1) diabetes, which requires insulin shots, appears to be more common in those who were vitamin D deficient as children. Type 1 diabetes usually starts in children between 8 and 12 years of age. It affects 15,000 to 100,000 children per year. Adults can also develop this type of diabetes. Type I diabetes results when the immune system attacks the beta cells of the pancreas, which are responsible for the production of insulin, a regulator of blood sugar. When a person is diagnosed with diabetes, physicians can do blood tests to help differentiate type 1 from type 2 diabetes.

A study by Elina Hyppönem, PhD (Centre for Paediatric Epidemiology and Biostatistics, Institute of Child Health, London), of 12,055 children in northern Finland born in 1966 showed that children who were supplemented with 2,000 IU/day of vitamin D during their first year of life were 78% chance less likely to develop type 1 (insulin dependent) diabetes from 1967 to 1997, when compared to those not supplemented. Stated another way, for every 10 children who developed diabetes, 8 could have been prevented if they had supplemented with vitamin D. In addition, those with rickets were 3 times more likely to develop type 1 diabetes. This study indicates the strong relationship between vitamin D supplementation during childhood and prevention of type 1 diabetes.

Another study by Lars C. Stene, PhD (National Institute of Public Health, Oslo, Norway) and colleagues concluded that cod liver oil and/or vitamin D supplementation by mothers during pregnancy reduced the risk of type 1 diabetes in their offspring.

Jon was a 13 year old boy who developed body aches and a flu-like illness. He quickly became dehydrated and severely ill. No matter how much water his parents gave him, he was unable to keep hydrated due to vomiting. His parents took him to the local emergency room. Doctors conducted blood tests and were surprised to learn that his blood sugar was over 500 mg/ml, normal is less than 100 mg/ml. Additional blood tests showed that his blood had a high level acid in it. Fortunately, aggressive intravenous (IV) fluids helped restore him back to normal after a few days. Additional testing showed that Jon was a type 1 diabetic. Jon would now require daily insulin shots for the rest of his life. His new way of living would be a challenge to the entire family. As I think back to my encounters with Jon and his family, I wonder if vitamin D deficiency contributed to his diabetes? If his mom had supplemented with cod liver oil and vitamin D could this have been prevented?

I would recommend that you have your child's vitamin D level checked the next time you go to the doctor. Most doctors check a child's hemoglobin level at ages 1 to 3. In addition, physicians are now encouraged to check cholesterol levels in at-risk children. The next time your child goes for a physical exam, ask your doctor to do a vitamin D blood test.

Type 2 Diabetes Mellitus

Diabetes is a serious problem in the U.S. and worldwide. In the U.S. alone, 24 million adults and children have diabetes, according to the American Diabetes Association. Unfortunately, 25% of them are not yet aware of their diabetes. Poor access to quality health care is partly to blame. An estimated 150 million people worldwide have diabetes. That number could double to 300 million by 2030. As Americans, Europeans, Asians, and others become fatter, the incidence of diabetes will increase. If the current trend continues, it is now predicted that 1 in 2 children born today will become diabetic as an adult. The main cause of this is obesity, poor diet, and inactivity.

Studies show that vitamin D could also be involved. Several studies have shown a relationship between vitamin D status and risks of developing both type 1 and type 2 diabetes. Below, I have cited some of the studies that support this.

Anastassios G. Pittas, MD (Tufts-New England Medical Center, Boston, MA), and colleagues published a study in *Diabetes Care*. They studied 83,779 women from the Nurse's Health Study and showed that those who took 1,200 mg of calcium with 800 IU of vitamin D had a 33% reduction in developing diabetes compared to those who took half as much. Dr. Pittas' study also showed that supplementation of vitamin D was more important than simply getting it through food, which is a poor source of vitamin D. Also, his study showed that the benefits from taking calcium and vitamin D were better than simply taking vitamin D alone.

> **"This study showed that Caucasians and Mexican-Americans with the highest levels of vitamin D were 75% and 83%, respectively, less likely to be diabetic when compared to those with the lowest blood levels of vitamin D"**

A study by Robert Scragg, PhD (School of Population Health, University of Auckland, New Zealand), and colleagues published in *Diabetes Care* also showed significant results. This study showed that Caucasians and Mexican-Americans with the highest levels of vitamin D were 75% and 83%, respectively, less likely to be diabetic when compared to those with the lowest blood levels of vitamin D. In essence, high vitamin D blood levels strongly protected at risk populations from developing diabetes. Mexican-Americans have some of the highest rates of diabetes of any ethnic group in the USA.

Debra Blair, MPH, RD (Fresenius Medical Care, Western Massachusetts Kidney Center, Springfield, Massachusetts), and colleagues published a study in the *Journal of Renal Nutrition, 2008*. The study evaluated diabetes control in those with advanced kidney failure. Researchers found that 80% of those with failure had vitamin D deficient levels below 31 ng/ml (77 nmol/L). These diabetic patients were then supplemented with 50,000 IU of vitamin D2 once a week and saw their hemoglobin A1C (HgA1C), a marker for diabetes control, improve by 0.5% (from 6.9% to 6.4%), indicating a significant improvement in their blood sugars.

Medicines such as pioglitazone (Actos®), which is used to control diabetes, can expect to produce a 0.9% to 1.9% decrease in HgA1C. Simply stated, vitamin D when optimized may be about 25% to 50% as effective as prescription diabetic medicines, at a fraction of the cost. Talk to your doctor before making any changes to your diabetes regimen. Whether these benefits will apply to those diabetics without advanced kidney disease is unknown at this time; however, future research and scientific studies will help answer the question.

Diabetes, when diagnosed, is usually treated with diet and exercise. In addition, the following pills help control diabetes.

- Biguanides- Metformin (Glucophage®) helps to make muscle cells more sensitive to the effects of insulin
- Sulfonylureas- Glipizide (Glucotrol®), glyburide (Micronase®) and glimepiride (Amaryl®) stimulate the pancreas to make more insulin
- Thiazolidinediones- Pioglitazone (Actos®) and rosiglitazone (Avandia®) work to help make insulin more effective
- DPP-4 Inhibitors- Sitalgliptin (Januvia®) works by increasing insulin and decreasing liver production of sugar.

When the above medications do not control blood sugar sufficiently, a person may require insulin injections. Diabetes medicines should never be stopped unless directed by a physician. Vitamin D does not interact with any diabetic medicines.

Not all studies showed protection of vitamin D against diabetes. A study by Ian H. de Boer, MD (University of Washington, Seattle, Washington), and colleagues evaluated 33,951 postmenopausal women without diabetes who were randomly assigned to take 1,000 mg of calcium and 400 IU of vitamin D, or a placebo. These women were followed for 7 years. The study concluded, "Calcium plus vitamin D supplementation did not reduce the risk of developing diabetes over 7 years of follow-up in this randomized placebo-controlled trial."

However the authors went on to suggest that perhaps higher levels of vitamin D were needed, as supported by Dr. Pittas' study and others. It is clear that the 400 IU of vitamin D, found in most over-the-counter supplements, is ineffective. If you are taking an over-the-counter multivitamin, make sure you are getting a total of 2,000 IU of vitamin D daily. You will likely need to take an additional vitamin D supplement for this to occur. Ask your physician to measure your blood levels.

To summarize, the evidence is conclusive that vitamin D deficiency is common in all diabetics, both type 1 and type 2, and that the presence of a deficiency in childhood appears to increases one's risk of developing type 1 diabetes. In addition, vitamin D deficiency also appears to increase risk of developing type 2 diabetes. If you, or a family member, are a diabetic, it is vital that you ask your physician to evaluate your vitamin D level. Supplementing with at least 2,000 IU or possibly more may be required to elevate vitamin D levels above 50 ng/ml (125 nmol/L).

Diet and exercise can help control blood sugar in insulin-dependent type 1 diabetics and type 2 diabetics. However, type 2 diabetics must not underestimate the role diet and exercise play in not only controlling but also reversing diabetes. It is important that those with diet-induced type 2 diabetes do not simply rely on pills to control their diabetes. Being active in controlling and reversing diabetes is vital if you are to prevent heart attacks, strokes, blindness, and kidney failure.

SECTION VI:
AUTOIMMUNE CONDITIONS

"The part can never be well unless the whole is well." - Plato

Multiple Sclerosis

Multiple sclerosis (MS) is a condition in which one's own immune system destroys the covering of the nerves. This is analogous to a mouse eating the plastic coating on an electrical wire—the result is a type of "short circuit" in the nerve. This short circuit results in numbness, tingling, and muscle weakness. According to the National Multiple Sclerosis Society, MS affects 1 in 700 people in the U.S., or almost 400,000 people overall.

The National Multiple Sclerosis Society defines MS as:

Multiple sclerosis (or MS) is a chronic, often disabling disease that attacks the central nervous system (CNS), which is made up of the brain, spinal cord, and optic nerves. Symptoms may be mild, such as numbness in the limbs, or severe, such as paralysis or loss of vision. The progress, severity, and specific symptoms of MS are unpredictable and vary from one person to another. Today, new treatments and advances in research are giving new hope to people affected by the disease.

Medical students have learned for years that those populations farther from the equator are at higher risk for MS than those living closer to the equator. We never understood why this was the case; we are only now beginning to understand the connection with vitamin D. Hundreds of research articles have appeared in journals, a few of which I discuss below.

In animal studies, treatment with vitamin D has prevented MS in treated groups.

In 2004, Kassandra L. Munger, MSc, (Harvard School of Public Health), and her colleagues published a study in *American Academy of Neurology*. The results showed that women with higher vitamin D intake were protected from developing MS compared to those with lower intake of vitamin D. The study reviewed diet and supplement habits of women in the Nurse's Health Study and the Nurse's Health Study II. In total, over 187,000 women were included and they were studied from 1980 to 2001. Those women who were in the top 20% of vitamin D consumption had a 33% reduction in MS when compared to those women with the lowest vitamin D intake in their diet. In addition, women who consumed greater than 400 IU or more of vitamin D through a supplement were 41% less likely to develop MS compared to those who did not take supplements.

> **"Those with vitamin D levels greater than 39 ng/ml (99 nmol/L) were 62% less likely to develop MS when compared to those with the lowest levels of vitamin D..."**

Another study by Kassandra L. Munger, MSc (Harvard School of Public Health) appeared in the *Journal of the American Medical Association (JAMA)* in 2006 with even more impressive results. Those with vitamin D levels greater than 39 ng/ml (99 nmol/L) were 62% less likely to develop MS when compared to those with the lowest levels of vitamin D circulating in their blood. This is a significant benefit. This information clearly explains why those who live closer to the equator, where there is more sunlight exposure, have lower rates of multiple sclerosis when compared to those in farther from the equator.

Another study by Jeri Nieves, PhD (Helen Hayes Hospital, West Haverstraw, NY) showed that a high percentage of women with MS have vitamin D deficiency. The study of 80 people with MS showed an average vitamin D blood level of 17 ng/ml (43 nmol/L). This is almost half the normal value of 32 ng/ml (80 nmol/L). The study also showed that 23% of these women were severely deficient, with levels less than 10 ng/ml (25 nmol/L). These women with MS also had extremely weak bones, leading researchers to conclude that these women with MS had a two to three times increased risk for bone fractures.

A European study by Dr. Barbara van Amerongen (VU Medical Center, Amsterdam, The Netherlands) concluded: "Optimal 25 OH-D (Vitamin D) serum concentrations, throughout the year, may be beneficial for patients with MS, both to obtain immune-mediated suppression of disease activity, and also to decrease disease-related complications, including increased bone resorption, fractures, and muscle weakness."

Numerous other studies show that vitamin D deficiency is extremely common in those with MS. Animal studies have supported aggressive treatment with vitamin D to help reverse numerous symptoms and complications of MS. This is a hot area of research and more studies are needed to see to what degree vitamin D optimization can not only prevent the development of MS, but also minimize the symptoms of those suffering with MS. In either case, those with MS or with a family history of it should contact their physicians about having a vitamin D blood test.

Rheumatoid Arthritis

Rheumatoid Arthritis (RA) is a systemic inflammatory condition that can affect various parts of the body. Generally, the joints are the primary targets and, when affected, can cause severe disability and pain. This dreaded disease usually occurs around the 3rd and 6th decades, and affects women twice as much as men. Overall, about 1 in 100 people are affected. In addition to affecting the joints, rheumatoid arthritis can affect the arteries, kidneys, nerves or even cause pericarditis, inflammation around the heart.

RA is autoimmune in nature, meaning that the body's own immune system inappropriately attacks its own cells, tissues, internal organs, and joints—leading to disease, inflammation, and pain. The mechanism is similar to the way in which the body's nerves are attacked in MS. The treatment for RA often includes steroid medications like prednisone and other immune system-lowering medications. As already seen, vitamin D deficiency seems to play a role in diseases and deficiencies of the immune system. In addition, several studies show that vitamin D deficiency is very common in those with RA.

A 2005 study by Graham Chiu, MD, reported in the *New Zealand Medical Journal* involved 55 patients with RA. Dr. Chiu showed that (78%) of those afflicted had vitamin D levels below 20 ng/ml (50 nmol/L); and 12 (22%) were severely deficient, with a level below 10 ng/ml (25 nmol/L). He went on to conclude that this vitamin D deficiency likely contributed to the musculoskeletal symptoms these patients experienced. When I further evaluated the data, only 3 patients (5%) had what we now consider a normal vitamin D serum level above 32 ng/ml (80 nmol/L). Stated another way, 95% of these patients with RA were vitamin D deficient.

A study reported by Diana Mahoney in *Family Practice News 2008* cited research by Dr. Uzzma Haque of Johns Hopkins University. Dr. Haque found that patients with RA who had vitamin D blood levels below 30 ng/ml (75 nmol/L) had more difficulty performing activities of daily living such as bathing, brushing teeth, and cooking when compared to those with levels above 30 ng/ml (75 nmol/L).

This is still a growing area of research and we need more studies before we can draw definitive conclusions. However, the preliminary results are encouraging. If you have rheumatoid arthritis, ask your primary physician or rheumatologist to order a vitamin D blood test. I recommend you attempt to get your levels above 50 ng/ml (125 nmol/L) for optimal pain relief and bone strengthening. In addition, it appears that the disability and the symptoms associated with RA may at least be minimized when blood levels are higher.

Lupus

Lupus, or Systemic Lupus Erythematosus (SLE) as it is sometimes referred to, is an autoimmune condition that affects various parts of the body. When lupus is present, the body's immune system (antibodies) attacks cells, tissues, and organs as it does in RA. Those with lupus have an inflammatory condition that can affect a single part of the body or numerous parts. Some have mild forms, while others have forms that are more lethal. Some, including children, can even develop strokes from lupus and its complications.

Lupus predominantly affects women compared to men by a ratio of 10 to 1, while affecting 1 in 5,000 people overall. Traditional risk factors for lupus include being African-American, Hispanic, Asian, or Native American. In addition, there appears to be a genetic component to some who develop lupus.

Recent research with animal models by Jacques M. Lemire, MD (Pediatric Nephrology, The University of Texas Medical School of Houston, Texas, USA), and colleagues supports the idea that vitamin D is a protective factor against developing lupus and in the treatment of lupus symptoms.

A study by Diane L. Kamen, MD (Medical University of South Carolina), regarding vitamin D and lupus concluded: "These results suggest vitamin D deficiency as a possible risk factor for SLE (lupus) and provide guidance for future studies looking at a potential role of vitamin D in the prevention and/or treatment of SLE."

Another study by Dr. A. M. Huisman (Department of Rheumatology, Saint Franciscus Gasthuis, Kleiweg Rotterdam, Netherlands) showed that vitamin D deficiency is very common in the lupus patients—with average bloods level under 20 ng/ml (50 nmol/L). Normal is above 32 ng/ml (75 nmol/L).

Some people with lupus may have some of the following signs and symptoms:

- Arthritis pains
- Fever
- Fatigue
- Weight loss
- Butterfly shaped rash on face
- Mouth ulcers
- Hair Loss
- Sun sensitivity
- Dry eyes
- Chest pains
- Muscle tenderness
- Stiffness of joints
- Kidney disease

When present, it is important to diagnose early to prevent long-term disability. Furthermore, ensuring adequate vitamin D levels is important for bone health and for prevention of osteopenia or osteoporosis.

According to a study by Rosalind Ramsey-Goldman, MD, DrPH (Northwestern University, Chicago, Illinois) and colleagues, bone fractures occur in about 12% of those with lupus, which is 5 times higher than in the general population. This higher risk was seen in those diagnosed at an older age and in those who used more steroid medicines to treat their lupus. Both older age and steroid medicine use are risk factors for bone thinning, so paying extra attention to bone strength is vital. As shown previously, supplementing with vitamin D and calcium is important in preventing the thinning of bones and, ultimately, fractures.

If you (or a family member) have lupus, make sure you know what your vitamin D blood level is. Ensuring maximal calcium absorption is crucial. While the research studies are sparse regarding vitamin D and lupus, it is certain that more will be published in upcoming years.

Psoriasis

Psoriasis comes from the Greek word, *psora*, meaning itchy. It is a skin disorder that causes mild to severe dry skin patches on the arms, trunk, scalp, and just about anywhere else on the body. Some with psoriasis can also develop pitting on their finger nails. Psoriasis results from the inability of skin cells to effectively regulate their division. The result is that they multiply excessively, leaving dry skin patches as evidence.

The diagnosis is primarily clinical, while blood tests can show an elevated sedimentation rate or elevated C-reactive protein (CRP), indicating systemic inflammation. Certain environmental and emotional stressors can trigger a flare-up of psoriasis. Obesity is also associated with psoriasis. There also appears to be a genetic predisposition to psoriasis as many with the condition have someone in the family who is also affected.

People with psoriasis have several therapeutic options or drug treatments available. First, keeping the skin adequately hydrated can help control mild to moderate cases. When that fails, use of steroid creams can be helpful. However, side effects can include thinning of skin, loss of pigmentation, or risk of skin infection. Some people with psoriasis feel a social stigma associated with their disease, so control of this disease is important, while minimizing negative effects from prescription medicines.

Vitamin D creams such as calcipotriene (Dovonex®) are also beneficial. Applied once or twice daily and used in conjunction with steroids, this cream can achieve better results. However, the benefits last only while the cream is in use.

Sunshine also helps control psoriasis. Specifically, UVB light therapy is effective. Many dermatologists have UVB light therapy "boxes" in their offices.

When these medicines don't do the job, many consider pills such as methotrexate, cyclosporine, acitretin, adalimumab (Humira®) or etanercept (Enbrel®). However, these medicines have the potential for serious side effects, such as life-threatening infections. As a result, the decision to take these is a serious one. These immune-modulating medicines should truly be a last resort.

It is curious to note that vitamin D creams have become a common treatment for psoriasis, whereas oral vitamin D and vitamin D analogues have not. Is there evidence that vitamin D pills are not effective? Not that I can determine. Topical creams simply have a financial advantage to developers; their patentability makes them a more lucrative business opportunity.

In 1985, Dr. S. Morimoto and Dr. Kumahara (Department of Medicine and Geriatrics, Osaka University Medical School, Japan) published a case report in which an 81-year old man with osteoporosis received a vitamin D pill as treatment. After 2 months, his psoriasis skin plaque had completely resolved. Thus began vitamin D treatment for psoriasis.

A second study by Dr. S. Morimoto (Department of Medicine and Geriatrics, Osaka University Medical School, Japan) 4 years later, published in *Archives of Dermatology*, treated 17 patients with an oral vitamin D. After 3 months, 13 patients saw improvement. There were no side effects from oral vitamin D therapy.

A 1989 study by Diana B. Holland, BSc, PhD (Department of Dermatology, The General Infirmary at Leeds, Greenford, U.K), of 15 people revealed that 10 patients who took vitamin D supplements showed improvement in their psoriasis. Seven showed complete resolution, while 3 showed almost complete resolution. Five experienced no benefit after 4 to 6 months.

A 1991 study by O.E. Araugo (College of Pharmacy, University of Florida, Gainesville) and colleagues showed that treatment with oral vitamin D pills showed moderate improvement in 24 of 35 patients with psoriasis. The researchers concluded that vitamin D analog pills might prove to be a promising treatment for psoriasis.

In another study by Professor Ellen L. Smith (Department of Physiology and Nutrition, Tufts University), 10 of 14 patients with moderate to severe psoriasis showed significant clearing of their psoriasis. The authors concluded that "these preliminary findings suggest that orally...administered 1,25-(OH)2-D3 (Vitamin D) can be a safe and effective alternative therapy for the treatment of psoriasis."

Lastly, a 2008 study in *American Journal Clinical Nutrition* showed that obese patients with moderate to severe psoriasis who lost weight had a better response to the cyclosporine medicine and a low-calorie diet than those who did not lose weight. The study did not measure vitamin D levels, but since obese people are 57% more likely to have lower vitamin D levels, it would be interesting to know if those who lost weight saw their vitamin D levels increase, thereby allowing their psoriasis to improve.

I am not claiming that vitamin D is the cure for psoriasis but there is ample evidence that those with psoriasis are at risk for vitamin D deficiency. Furthermore, treatment with vitamin D appears to benefit over half of those with psoriasis. Topical vitamin D creams are also of benefit. Since many with psoriasis have plaques on their arms, vitamin D production from the interaction of the sun and skin is limited. It is important that all people with psoriasis check their vitamin D blood levels and optimize supplementation so that blood levels are above 50 ng/ml (125 nmol/L). Ask your physician which treatment options are best for you.

SECTION VII:
CANCER

HISTORY OF CANCER

The word *cancer* comes from Middle English and dates back to 1350-1400 AD. It is also the same word we use in the zodiac symbol to represent a crab. A person born from June 21st to July 22nd is of this zodiac symbol. The word comes from the Greek equivalent. The first descriptions of cancer appear in ancient Egyptian writings.

The Edwin Smith Medical Papyrus, a medical textbook of sorts, from the 16th century BC, provides the earliest description of what we now call cancer. It describes eight cases of tumors or ulcers of the female breast. At the time, people recognized that there was no treatment for such. In addition, it appears the Egyptians were able to distinguish between benign (good) and malignant (bad) tumors. The Ebers Papyrus, of around the same time, also mentions cancer, recounting a "tumor against the god Xenus," it recommends, "do thou nothing there against."

Hippocrates (460–370 BC), the Greek physician and person we consider to be the "father of medicine," described cancer. He noticed that malignant tumors had blood vessels that surrounded it in a claw-like manner. He used the word *karkinos* (*crab* in Greek) to describe these tumors. This is the origin of our words carcinoma and cancer.

How Common Is Cancer?

Cancer is one of the scariest words in the English language, especially when describing a diagnosis for you or a family member. For many, it signifies death. For others, it implies a dismal future and a lot of hard work, with no guarantees of success. In the U.S. alone, it is estimated that there were 1,437,180 cases of cancer in 2008, resulting in 565,660 deaths or 1,549 deaths a day. Cancer is the No. 2 killer in America, second only to heart disease and stroke.

Cancer is also a big killer worldwide. According to the World Health Organization, in the year 2000, 12% of the world's 56 million deaths were due to cancer. Cancer killed 6.7 million people, a number close to the population of Hong Kong, China. What if we could cut that number in half with one simple intervention? Would that not be an amazing accomplishment? The World Health Organization also calculated that in 2000, 5.3 million men and 4.7 million women worldwide developed cancer, a number far too big to tolerate. Ten million citizens of the world developed cancer. That is equivalent to the persons in over 100 football stadiums (each holding 100,000 individuals) developing cancer.

Overall, the past 50 years have seen significant gains in the number of deaths prevented from all causes. The lifespan of Americans, Europeans, and many other nationalities is now at all-time highs. Over the past 5 decades, there have been 66% fewer heart disease deaths and strokes. This significant progress is likely because we now have treatments for diabetes, high blood pressure, and high cholesterol, all risk factors for heart-related deaths.

In addition, since the 1960s, the number of tobacco smokers in the U.S. has diminished from 40% of the population in 1965 to 20.8% in 2006. Due to advances in sanitation, antibiotics, and our knowledge of infectious diseases, we also see fewer people dying from common infections.

Unfortunately, we have seen only a small decline in the number of cancer-related deaths. This small decline is likely the result of the mass screening exams such as the colonoscopy, Pap smear, mammogram, and possibly the blood PSA test for prostate cancer. However, we still have a lot of work to do.

The American Cancer Society (ACS) and their Relay for Life gets local community members involved in the fight against cancer. The ACS helps raise money for scientific research. While there is still a lot of work to be done, the ACS is on the right tract. They have even funded some vitamin D

research studies. Fortunately, research funded from all arenas has demonstrated that mass vitamin D testing and supplementation can help reduce
the number of cancer cases by 20% to 70%, depending on the type. This is
a great step in the right direction.

The American Cancer Society provides the following estimates (Table 8)
for developing cancer in the U.S. in 2008. Men have a 50% chance of developing cancer of any site, while women have a 33% chance. These numbers
do not include nonmelanoma skin cancers (basal cell and squamous cell), as
they are not usually life-threatening. These statistics are troubling and action
needs to be taken to decrease these rates.

Table 8. Lifetime probability of developing cancer.

Men	Women
All sites 1 in 2	All sites 1 in 3
Prostate 1 in 6	Breast 1 in 8
Lung and bronchus 1 in 13	Lung & bronchus 1 in 16
Colon and rectum 1 in 18	Colon & rectum 1 in 19
Urinary bladder 1 in 27	Uterine corpus 1 in 41
Melanoma 1 in 41	Non-Hodgkin's lymphoma 1 in 53
Non-Hodgkin's lymphoma 1 in 46	Melanoma 1 in 61
Kidney 1 in 59	Ovary 1 in 71
Leukemia 1 in 67	Pancreas 1 in 76
Oral cavity 1 in 71	Urinary bladder 1 in 85
Stomach 1 in 88	Uterine cervix 1 in 142

Source: http://www.cancer.org/downloads/STT/2008CAFFfinalsecured.pdf

The American Cancer Society also estimated the number of U.S. deaths
from various cancers in 2008 (Table 9). Lung cancer is the number one
cause of cancer deaths, while breast, prostate, colon, ovary, and pancreatic
cancer follow. As you will see, vitamin D plays a role in the prevention and
treatment of many of these cancers.

| Table 9. American Cancer Society death estimates for 2008 in U.S. ||
Men (294,120 deaths)	Women (271,540 deaths)
Lung & bronchus 31%	Lung & bronchus 26%
Prostate 10%	Breast 15%
Colon & rectum 8%	Colon & rectum 9%
Pancreas 6%	Pancreas 6%
Liver & bile duct 4%	Ovary 6%
Leukemia 4%	Non-Hodgkin's lymphoma 6%
Esophagus 3%	Leukemia 3%
Non-Hodgkin's lymphoma 3%	Uterine corpus 3%
Kidney & renal pelvis 3%	Liver & bile duct 2%
All other sites 24%	Brain/other neurological cancer 2%
	All other sites 25%

Source: American Cancer Society Statistics. Excludes basal and squamous cell skin cancers. http://www.cancer.org/downloads/stt/CFF2008M&F_Sites.pdf

Did you know that you have cancer cells growing in your body right now? Don't worry; everyone has cancer cells present at any given time. Fortunately, for most, the immune system recognizes these abnormal cells and destroys them before they can grow uncontrollably. A cancer cell is simply a cell in the body that has lost the ability to stop multiplying itself. As a result, the cell keeps growing and growing, becoming a large mass of cells, referred to as a tumor.

How Cancer Affects People Differently

There are still many racial disparities when is comes to cancer. African-American males are 1.4 times more likely to get cancer of any site when compared to white American males. However, certain cancers, such as prostate cancer (2.4 times) and stomach cancer (2.3 times) are exceedingly more common in African-American males than white males. Studies have shown that even when controlled for health care insurance, access to care, and other variables, black males have higher rates of these cancers. This has lead many researchers to conclude that vitamin D could be the missing factor that predisposes certain ethnic populations to higher rates of cancer. The evidence also shows that blood levels of vitamin D are lower in African-American males compared to white males.

African-American women share this trend when compared to white women. African-American women have a 20% higher incidence of all cancers, while breast and colon cancer are 40% more common, stomach cancer is 120% more common, and uterine/cervical cancer is 110% more common in black women compared to white women. This fact should encourage all people, especially those with darker pigmentation, to check their vitamin D levels.

Emotional and Financial Costs of Cancer

What would you pay to live cancer free? One hundred dollars? One million dollars? The costs of cancer to our society are enormous. While the mental, emotional, and physical costs are priceless, the financial costs approached $220 billion dollars in 2007 alone, according to the National Institutes of Health. The breakdown appears below.

Direct Medical Costs: $89 billion (total of all health expenditures)

Indirect Morbidity Costs: $18.2 billion (cost of lost productivity due to illness)

Indirect Mortality Costs: $112 billion (cost of lost productivity due to premature death)

Source: http://www.cancer.org/docroot/MIT/content/MIT_3_2X_Costs_of_Cancer.asp

A 2007 Associated Press report estimated that simply waiting for cancer treatments and tests cost around $2.3 billion dollars annually. This included waiting for CT scans, sitting in doctors' waiting rooms, and simply watching medicine drip into the veins.

Since 2004, hundreds of published studies have shown the health benefits of vitamin D. They have shown that higher vitamin D blood levels can help prevent cancer and cancer recurrence. Whether obtaining vitamin D from food, sunlight, or supplementation, the overall results are favorable with no side effects.

A study funded by the American Cancer Society and published in 2002 shows the importance of sunlight exposure. William Grant, PhD (Director of the Sunlight, Nutrition, and Health Research Center, San Francisco), concluded:

The results of the current study demonstrate that much of the geographic variation in cancer mortality (death) rates in the U.S. can be attributed to variations in solar UV-B radiation (sunlight) exposure. Thus, many lives could be extended through increased careful exposure to solar UV-B radiation (sunlight) and more safely, vitamin D3 supplementation, especially in non summer months.

The study showed a reduction in the following cancers for those with higher exposure to sunlight:

- Bladder
- Esophageal
- Kidney
- Lung
- Pancreatic
- Rectal
- Stomach
- Uterine

To put it simply, if one lives in a state or country with a lot of sunshine, the likelihood of developing cancer is lower.

A 2002 study by Dr. Michael Freedman (National Cancer Institute) and colleagues published in *Occupational and Environmental Medicine* also concluded that people with more exposure to sunlight were less likely to die from breast cancer, ovarian cancer, prostate cancer, and colon cancer.

A study by Dr. Stefan Pilz and colleagues (Department of Public Health, Social and Preventive Medicine, Mannheim Medical Faculty, University of Heidelberg) concluded that low levels of vitamin D are associated with increased risk of fatal cancer. Maintenance of sufficient levels of vitamin D in the blood can help in the prevention and treatment of cancers.

As you will see below, numerous studies provide evidence of cancer prevention with vitamin D. Every person who is able should have his or her blood levels of vitamin D checked. I will review some of the deadliest cancers and the effect that vitamin D has on them. We will discuss cancers of the lung, breast, prostate, colon, cervix, ovary, and pancreas. In addition, we will discuss the correlation between vitamin D and skin melanoma.

Lung Cancer

Lung cancer is the No.1 cancer killer of both men and women in America. It accounts for 31% of all cancers in men and 26% of all cancers in women. One in 13 men will develop lung cancer while one in 16 women will develop it. Risk factors for lung cancer include: cigarette smoking, second hand smoke exposure, asbestos exposure, radon, air pollution and environmental toxins. Of these, cigarette smoke is the most dangerous. According to the CDC, up to 90% of lung cancers in men and 80% of all lung cancers in women are primarily due to cigarette smoking. In fact, cigarettes are responsible for over 1,200 deaths every day in the U.S. alone. In addition to lung cancer, cigarette smokers have increased risk for heart attacks and strokes, the No. 1 and No. 3 killers, respectively.

It is my recommendation that all smokers quit. If they don't, they should take vitamin D supplements and increase sunlight exposure. Vitamin D supplementation has numerous health benefits and could actually help prevent cancer from forming in the first place. It is important that smokers do not embrace a false sense of security by thinking that they can continue smoking since vitamin D will "prevent" them from getting cancer. However, it will at least decrease the number of smokers who die from lung cancer. Here is the evidence.

A 2008 study by Sharif B. Mohr, MPH (Department of Family and Preventive Medicine, University of California, San Diego), and colleagues studied the association of latitude and UV light exposure with lung cancer rates in 111 countries. The authors of the study concluded: "Lower levels of UVB irradiance (or sunlight) were independently associated with higher incidence rates of lung cancer in 111 countries." Basically, those countries with less sunlight exposure had higher rates of lung cancer, demonstrating the health and protective benefits of sunshine and vitamin D.

A 2005 study by Wei Zhou, MD, PhD (Occupational Health Program, Occupational Health Program, Harvard School of Public Health), and colleagues studied 456 patients with early stage (non-small cell) lung cancer. Researchers showed that patients who had surgery for their cancer in the summer, when vitamin D levels were higher, had a 53% chance of being cancer free at 5 years. Those who had surgery during the winter, when vitamin D blood levels are lower, had a 40% chance of survival at 5 years.

> **"Patients with early stage (non-small cell) lung cancer were 2 times more likely to be alive if they had higher vitamin D levels"**

Further analysis showed that cancer patients with the highest intake of vitamin D and summer surgery for their cancer had a 56% chance of survival, while those with the lowest vitamin D intake and surgery in the winter had only a 23% chance of survival at 5 years. In other words, this study showed that patients with early stage (non-small cell) lung cancer were 2 times more likely to be alive if they had higher vitamin D levels.

Also, a study by Trude Robsahm, MSc (Senior researcher at The Cancer Registry of Norway), showed that patients with breast, colon, and prostate cancer diagnosed and treated during the summer and fall—when vitamin D levels are higher—were less likely to die from their cancer than those diagnosed and treated in the winter or spring, when vitamin D levels are lower.

As vitamin D research continues to grow, it is certain that more studies will be done showing the relationship between sunlight, vitamin D, and lung cancer. These initial study results are encouraging. However, we also know that if a smoker quits, he or she can significantly decrease the risk of developing lung cancer and emphysema, regardless of how many years the person has smoked. My recommendation is to quit smoking and increase your sunlight exposure and vitamin D blood levels. If you don't smoke, encourage those you know who do smoke to quit. In addition to hypnosis, nicotine patches, and nicotine gum, there are now quality medicines available that can help smokers quit. Ask your doctor about Chantix, a medicine which appears to help up to 50% of its users to quit smoking. Also, don't forget to ask your doctor to check your vitamin D blood level.

Breast Cancer

According to statistics, breast cancer will affect one in eight women during their lifetime. In 2008, the American Cancer Society estimated that 40,731 women died from this dreaded disease. Breast cancer is one of the most frightening cancers a woman can have. The mammary glands represent life and hope to a newborn child, while also offering many women a sense of sex appeal. Many women strive to have more perfect breasts. Unfortunately, mass media—especially the movie and magazine industry—has created a false sense of inadequacy among many women who perhaps would never have thought they had a problem in the first place. This is evident by the fact that cosmetic breast augmentation surgery has become a billion dollar industry. Many women who have had augmentation feel a sense of empowerment, while some others have experienced medical problems. The following risk factors increase the likelihood of developing breast cancer.

- Older Age
- Family history
- Alcohol intake greater than 1 drink per day
- Being overweight or obese
- Increased breast density
- Hormonal exposure
- Ionizing radiation
- Lack of exercise
- Vitamin D deficiency

Of these risk factors, maintaining a healthy weight and exercising more can help reduce one's risk of breast cancer. While cancer of the breasts generally affects women over 35 years of age, those under 35 are not immune. I will share two experiences from my life where breast cancer directly affected my family and me. Experiences like these have inspired me to promote cancer prevention.

In 1998, my cousin Cathy was diagnosed with breast cancer. She and I used to play together as young children; my mom and her mom were sisters. We were only 6 months apart, to the day. She was a cute child who loved life. She and her family moved to Washington State, a state with more cloud covered days than sunny days. Shortly after graduating from high school, she got married. She and her husband had four children. Like any young couple, they had big plans for their future—plans to raise their children, live life, and enjoy each day to the fullest.

When I heard of her diagnosis, I was in the middle of medical school. She was 1,500 miles away in Washington State. While I was facing the rigors of medical education, my cousin and the rest of the family had a different battle to face—a life-or-death battle. There was little I could do as I was just learning about breast cancer. She fought the cancer and its attempt to take control of her body for years. She had surgery, chemotherapy, and radiation—the standard of care for breast cancer.

She had an amazingly strong will to survive. She knew she had to fight as hard as she could; she had four beautiful children who depended on her and needed their mommy to be there for them. She wondered if she would live to see them grow up, graduate from high school, and have families of their own. Would she live to see her grandchildren or would she even live to see another day?

In spite of the excellent medical care she received, her body did not respond. The cancer took over and spread throughout her body—first to her brain and then her spine, leaving her listless and bedbound. This once independent woman who cared for her husband and children now required them to care for her every need. There was little more that the cancer experts could do.

At the young age of 29, Cathy passed away, survived by her husband and four children, all under age 10. Surely, there was something that could have been done to help prevent this. While it was too late for my cousin Cathy, perhaps there is something out there that can help her younger sister,

Christine, prevent cancer. While family history is an important risk factor, whether or not those genes are turned on depends on diet, lifestyle, and environment.

The research shows that vitamin D also represents an important piece of the prevention puzzle. Did the fact that state of Washington has more days of rain than sunshine play a roll? I believe it did. As we will see, there are numerous research studies to show the protective benefits of vitamin D and sunshine against breast cancer.

In addition, my stepmother, Dori, learned that she had breast cancer at the young age of 27. She spent little time sunbathing, in spite of living in California. She received the standard surgery and radiation therapy. While she considered alternative treatments, she was skeptical; she had a friend who had visited an alternative medicine practitioner in Mexico, was treated with apricot seeds (which have laetrile in them, an alternative cancer treatment used by some), and died shortly thereafter. Fortunately, Dori was able to fight the cancer off and is today doing well. She is now a 28-year survivor, and counting.

My concern now is to make sure that my sister Lauren, who is 25 years old, prevents cancer in the first place. She goes to her yearly doctor exams, eats healthy foods, exercises, and takes her vitamin D. All these lifestyle behaviors can help prevent cancer from ever occurring. Even if there is a genetic risk, Lauren's wise actions can keep the cancer genes turned off, while turning on the longevity genes.

I recently came across a report of a 21-year old woman who was diagnosed with breast cancer. Fortunately, she was also able to survive it. She had great support from her friends and family. However, for a young person who is just beginning her life, she has already had to face major life-changing challenges.

While there are many reasons some people defeat cancer and others don't, living a healthy lifestyle is paramount, especially after cancer is diagnosed. Even that will not guarantee anything, but it will significantly increase your odds of surviving. While the examples I discussed were of women under 30, most breast cancers affect those over 40 years of age.

"Experts recommend that all women have their first mammogram at age 40, then every 1 or 2 years thereafter"

Breast cancer is usually first identified when a woman, or her doctor, notices a lump growing on the breast that did not exist before. Experts recommend that all women have their first mammogram at age 40, then every 1 or 2 years thereafter. For women 50 or older, doctors recommend a yearly mammogram. For women at higher risk for breast cancer, physicians may recommend mammogram screening at a younger age or breast MRIs. It is important for a woman to talk to her family doctor or gynecologist to see what recommendation is best for her.

A woman who has never had one may wonder what a mammogram is. A mammogram is an X-ray of the breast that helps detect an existing breast cancer. Many women loathe having one, as the breasts are often "squished" during the X-ray. While having a mammogram is very important because early detection can help prevent dying from breast cancer, a mammogram does not prevent breast cancer. It detects cancer once it is already there. As technology improves, MRIs will be used more frequently for the detection of breast cancers, as they might detect them at earlier stages. Perhaps we will eventually have a blood test to help detect breast cancer.

As a family doctor, I would rather prevent 100 women from ever developing breast cancer in the first place than detect breast cancer in the same 100 women. This stresses the importance of primary care and preventive medicine. In addition, it is important that women perform monthly breast exams in order to alert their physicians of any changes that they notice. Physicians don't expect a woman to differentiate a *bad* lump from a *good* lump, simply to recognize any changes in the breast since any prior exam.

Research has shown that healthy diets, such as those low in saturated fats (red meats, cheese, and dairy) and high in fruits and vegetables, have a beneficial effect on breast cancer prevention. In addition, maintaining a healthy body weight and exercising regularly can help prevent breast cancer.

A 2006 study by researcher Martin Lajous (Center for Population Health Research, Cuernavaca, Mexico) and colleagues from Harvard Medical School supports this. Researchers showed that diets high in fruits and vegetables are protective against many cancers, and studies have shown that high intake of folic acid and vitamin B12 is also associated with decreased breast cancer, especially among postmenopausal women.

While antioxidants such as vitamins C and E have many benefits to overall health, a recent study by Eunyoung Cho, ScD (Harvard Medical School), and colleagues showed that these vitamins were not protective against breast cancer when taken early in life. However, there is also no evidence of their being harmful.

Having dense breasts is also a risk factor for breast cancer. Those women with denser breasts are five times more likely to get breast cancer compared to those with less dense breasts. However, several studies, including a 2004 study by Sylvie Bérubé, MSc (Centre des maladies du sein Deschênes-Fabia, Centre hospitalier affilié universitaire de Québec, Quebec, Canada), have shown that those women with higher intakes of calcium and vitamin D have lower breast tissue density, which ultimately lowers the risk of breast cancer.

A study by Jacques Brisson, PhD (University Laval, Quebec, Canada), published in 2007 evaluated 741 premenopausal women. The researchers concluded that seasonal changes in vitamin D seem to be inversely related to changes in breast density. Further, the scientists stated the possibility that vitamin D could reduce breast density and breast cancer risk should encourage further investigation.

Another study by Sylvie Bérubé, MSc, and colleagues in 2005, concluded that when premenopausal women had high intakes of vitamin D and calcium from food sources and supplements, they had less dense breasts and, therefore, a reduced risk for breast cancer. The researchers went on to state, "increasing intakes of vitamin D and calcium may represent a safe and inexpensive strategy for breast cancer prevention".

Further, many women think that, because a family member had breast cancer, they are destined for the same. However, it is important to realize that genes, such as BRCA 1 and BRCA 2 (breast cancer genes), need to be turned on before they can cause problems. While a person can have the gene for breast cancer, poor diet, lack of exercise, or environmental exposures can actually be the key that turns that gene on, resulting in cancer cells having the opportunity to grow.

The good news is that vitamin D supplementation and increased sunshine exposure offer preventive effects against breast cancer development. This is an inexpensive way to ensure health and longevity. While integrating all the preventive measures together is ideal, having elevated vitamin D levels significantly reduces your chance of developing breast cancer. Spending adequate time in the sun and/or taking a vitamin D supplement can literally help save your life.

In a 1990 study, of people in the former Soviet Union, Edward D. Gorham, MPH, PhD (Department of Community and Family Medicine, University of California, San Diego, School of Medicine), reported lower rates of breast cancer in areas where there was more solar radiation, a consequence of more sunlight exposure. In his study, he also cited findings that countries within 20° of the equator have a lower incidence of breast cancer, compared to areas farther from the equator. This supports the notion that less sunshine results in less vitamin D generation and, ultimately, results in higher breast cancer rates.

In a 2002 study, Dr. Michael Freedman (National Cancer Institute) and his colleagues reported results that showed those who lived in areas with more sunshine exposure, or had jobs with more sunlight exposure, were 17% less likely to die from breast cancer, independent of their physical activity levels.

A study by Julia A. Knight, PhD (Prosserman Centre for Health Research, Mount Sinai Hospital, Toronto, Canada), of over 2,000 women showed that increased sun exposure as a young woman could prevent breast cancer later in life. Specifically, those girls getting more sun exposure from ages 10 to 19 reduced breast cancer by 35%, and those using regular cod liver oil reduced risk of breast cancer by 24%. Again, take caution; serious sunburns before the age of 18 have been associated with increased risk of skin cancers.

These studies show strong evidence of the health benefits of sunshine in preventing cancer. So many people have been trying to avoid the sun in an attempt to prevent skin cancer that it is possible we may have actually been putting ourselves at risk for more deadly cancers. Vitamin D supplementation also has favorable effects.

> **"A 2007 study by Cedric F. Garland... showed a 50% reduction in breast cancer in women who had vitamin D levels greater than 52 ng/ml (130 nmol/L)..."**

In a study by Kim Robien, PhD (Division of Epidemiology and Community Health, University of Minnesota School of Public Health), and colleagues studied 34,321 women who responded to questionnaires about diet and vitamin D supplement use. The women were followed from 1986 to 2004. Women who consumed more than 800 IU/day were compared to those who ingested less than 400 IU/day of vitamin D. The results showed an 11% reduction in breast cancer in those who consumed more vitamin D. However, during the first 5 years, results showed a 34% reduction in breast cancer incidence.

The researchers concluded that, over time, those who took more vitamin D could have decreased their intake, resulting in decreased benefits as years went on. Interestingly, most foods and over- the-counter vitamins used to have the less potent vitamin D2 (ergocalciferol), instead of the vitamin D3 (cholecalciferol) that is now used. So the results may have been less than maximal.

A 2005 study by Elizabeth R. Bertone-Johnson, ScD (Department of Public Health, University of Massachusetts), and colleagues showed that women over 60 years of age who had vitamin D blood levels above 40 ng/ml (100 nmol/L) compared to women with levels below 20 ng/ml (50 nmol/L), had a 43% reduction in breast cancer. The researchers concluded that high levels of vitamin D are modestly associated with a reduced risk of breast cancer.

Furthermore, a 2007 study by Cedric F. Garland, DrPH (Moores Cancer Center, University of California, San Diego) and colleagues of 1,760 women showed a 50% reduction in breast cancer in women who had vitamin D levels greater than 52 ng/ml (130 nmol/L), when compared to women who had levels below 13 ng/ml (32.5 nmol/L). The researchers concluded that a level of 52 ng/ml (130 nmol/L) could be achieved by supplementing with 2,000 IU of vitamin D daily and spending approximately 12 minutes per day in the sun. Ask your doctor to check your vitamin D level so you know where you are and where you need to be to obtain this great benefit.

> **"Those women who lived in geographic areas with more sunlight exposure, and therefore more solar radiation exposure, had a 25% to 65% reduction in breast cancer"**

Lastly, Esther M. John, PhD (Northern California Cancer Center), and her colleagues analyzed data collected over 20 years that showed some significant findings. Altogether, 5,009 women in the U.S. participated. The researchers found that higher sunlight exposure and increased dietary intake of vitamin D were associated with a 15% to 33% reduction in breast cancer. In addition, those women who lived in geographic areas with more sunlight exposure, and therefore more solar radiation exposure, had a 25% to 65% reduction in breast cancer.

The evidence is clear; you can significantly reduce your risk of developing breast cancer with no side effects. Increase your exposure to the sun, supplement your diet with vitamin D, and have your vitamin D blood levels checked. It's sad that few have heard this lifesaving news.

Gene Therapy and Breast Cancer

Those women who have developed or have inherited genetic mutations of the BRCA1 and BRCA2 genes are at increased risk for breast cancer. When these genes are functioning normally, they act to suppress breast cancer from developing. Breast cancer and the genetics of it have become a popular area for researchers. Scientists have learned that certain types of breast cancer are more sensitive to hormones, such as estrogen.

There is also a lot of research being conducted on vitamin D receptors, which are present in the tissues of most cancer cells. A Google Scholar search in early 2009 of scientific articles on "vitamin D receptors" yielded over 1,200 scientific studies since 2005 and over 4,500 studies since 1990. As scientists learn more about vitamin D receptors (VDRs) and the genetics of them, gene therapy that uses the pathways of VDRs could become a new route for medicines or vitamin D to prevent and treat cancers in the future.

A study by Wendy Y. Chen, MD, MPH (Instructor in Medicine, Harvard Medical School & Dana Farber Cancer Institute), concluded, "VDRs may be a mediator of breast cancer risk and could represent a target for cancer prevention efforts."This area of cancer research will prove to be a vital area in the future.

An additional study by Dr. Kristina M. Blackmore (Samuel Lunenfeld Research Institute, Mount Sinai Hospital, Toronto, Ontario, Canada) and colleagues evaluated almost 1,900 women and concluded that, "Vitamin D is associated with reduced risk of breast cancer regardless of estrogen/progesterone receptor status of the tumor."

In other words, whether there was a hormone influence on the cancer really did not matter; vitamin D was protective. This is important for women who are on medicines like tamoxifen (Soltamaox®) or raloxifene (Evista®), designed to reduce risk of recurrent breast cancer by minimizing the effects of the body's estrogen on breast tissue that is sensitive to hormones. Interestingly, women also take these medicines for osteoporosis, and the manufacturers recommend that women who take it for that purpose take calcium and a vitamin D supplement to help strengthen their bones.

What if a woman already has breast cancer? Is there any benefit to optimizing her vitamin D level? While there are few studies on this, a study conducted in Norway by Trude Robsahm, MSc (Senior researcher at The Cancer Registry of Norway), showed that those diagnosed with breast cancer during the summer and fall, when vitamin D blood levels are higher, had better prognoses than those diagnosed in the winter and spring. Similar results occurred for prostate and colon cancer.

To summarize, if you are a woman, you are at quite significant risk for breast cancer. Making healthier choices, becoming more physically active, and eating organic fruits and vegetables can significantly reduce your risk of ever developing breast cancer. However, one simple intervention can markedly reduce your risk of developing breast cancer—elevate your blood vitamin D levels. This can easily be done with vitamin D supplementation and increased sun exposure.

Don't assume that your multivitamin is providing you enough vitamin D, as they rarely do. You need to contact your physician, and ask him or her to check your vitamin D level. If your levels are below 50 ng/ml (125 ng/ml), start supplementing with at least 2,000 IU daily of vitamin D and recheck your blood levels in 3 months. It is important that you share this book with every woman you know, as that decision will ultimately become a lifesaving one. Together, we can help prevent breast cancer in revolutionary ways.

Colon Cancer

Colon cancer is one of the top three cancers affecting those in developed countries. According to the American Cancer Society, colon cancer accounts for 8% of all cancer deaths in men and 9% of all cancer deaths in women in the U.S. Colon cancer will affect 1 in 18 men and 1 in 19 women at some point in their lives. Fortunately, the majority of cases can be prevented. Worldwide, the World Health Organization predicts that colon cancer rates will increase 50% by 2020 and will affect up to 20 million people annually.

Risk factors for developing colon cancer include:

- Colon Polyps
- Poor diet, especially high in red meats
- Overweight
- Obesity
- Racial Groups (African Americans & Ashkenazi Jews)
- Lack of exercise
- Excess alcohol intake
- Family history
- Type 2 diabetes
- Vitamin D deficiency

Those with higher consumption of fruits and vegetables have a benefit in preventing colon cancer from developing in the first place. A 1996 study reported in *JAMA* suggested that the trace mineral selenium, a potent antioxidant, and part of the glutathione reductase antioxidant complex, could also be protective against precancerous polyps and colon cancer.

There has been renewed interest in the last few years on the ability of sunshine to prevent colon cancer. Specifically, the sunshine vitamin has anti colon cancer properties, observed back in the 1930s, and later confirmed in the 1980s by Cedric Garland, DrPH (Moores Cancer Center University of

California, San Diego), and Frank C. Garland, PhD, FACE (Technical Director, Naval Health Research Center (NHRC), San Diego).

Drs. Cedric and Frank Garlands' landmark study showed that the risk of colon cancer was associated with solar radiation exposure; many other studies have since confirmed this finding. Drs. Garlands' 1980 study revealed that in the two states with the most solar radiation, New Mexico and Arizona, white males had cancer rates of 6.7 and 10.1, respectively, per 100,000 people. In the three states with the least solar radiation, New York, Vermont, and New Hampshire, white males experienced colon cancer rates of 17.3, 11.3, and 15.3, respectively, per 100,000 population. Data collection occurred from 1959 to 1961. The conclusion was that those with more sunshine exposure had less colon cancer when compared to those with less sunshine exposure.

A review of the CDC web site and the statistics for colon and rectal cancer from 2002–2004 shows similar results. The data today is more inclusive, with men and women from all ethnicities. Arizona and New Mexico have total colon and rectal cancer rates of 49.9 and 51.8, respectively, per 100,000 population. On the contrary, New York, Vermont, and New Hampshire have rates of 63.0, 57.9, and 59.9, respectively, per 100,000 population.

However, note that there are definitely other factors that can predispose one to colon cancer. This is evident by the fact that the southern state of Louisiana has a rate of 69.1 cases per 100,000, while the northern state of Wyoming shows a rate of 49.0. Perhaps dietary habits and the larger African-American population in the state of Louisiana, a group that traditionally has lower vitamin D, factor into these results.

The American Cancer Society and other leading professional organizations recommend that all average-risk people be screened for colon cancer starting at age 50. This simple act appears to reduce colon cancer incidence. Certain polyps in the colon can put people at risk for colon cancer. Benign (noncancerous) hyperplastic polyps generally have no risk of becoming cancer, while adenomatous polyps can become cancer and, if found, must be removed. Adenomatous polyps are premalignant (precancerous) polyps and can take 5 to 7 years to develop into colon cancer (adenocarcinoma). Therefore, adenomatous polyps need close follow-up and possibly a repeat colonoscopy in 3 to 5 years, depending on their size and number.

- Colon cancer screening should begin at age 50 for most people in the form of a colonoscopy, sigmoidoscopy, or fecal occult stool testing.
- Those with first-degree relatives (a mom, a dad, or siblings) should be screened 10 years earlier than the age at which the relative was diagnosed with colon cancer.

If your mom, dad, or sibling had colon cancer, you should be screened 10 years earlier than the age at which your relative was diagnosed with the colon cancer. In other words, if your parent had colon cancer at age 50, then you should have a colonoscopy at age 40.

For those individuals with no symptoms and no family history of colon cancer, screening options at age 50 can include a sigmoidoscopy, colonoscopy, or simply screening with occult blood stool cards. Ask your physician which test is best for you.

Digestive System

To understand why cancer of the digestive system (Figure 10) can develop, it is important to understand how the digestive system works. When a person eats food, it goes through several stages before the body excretes the waste byproducts.

1. When you chew food, it mixes with saliva, which has digestive enzymes and helps initiate the breakdown of the food.
2. Food then goes down the esophagus, the hollow tube that connects the mouth to the stomach.
3. Food enters the stomach, where enzymes and stomach acids digest it more. This breaks the food down into smaller molecules.
4. Food enters the small intestine (the three parts include: duodenum, jejunum, ileum), which is the area where the majority of the nutrients are extracted. The gallbladder releases bile, which helps absorb fats, and the pancreas releases additional enzymes, which help the body absorb nutrients into the bloodstream so muscles, the brain, and the heart can utilize the nutrients for energy.

5. Food waste, which is essentially absent of nutrients, passes into the large intestine, or colon (ascending, transverse, descending and sigmoid colon), where water is absorbed and the formation of stool occurs. If the water is not absorbed, a person has diarrhea. The large intestine is where colon cancer frequently forms.

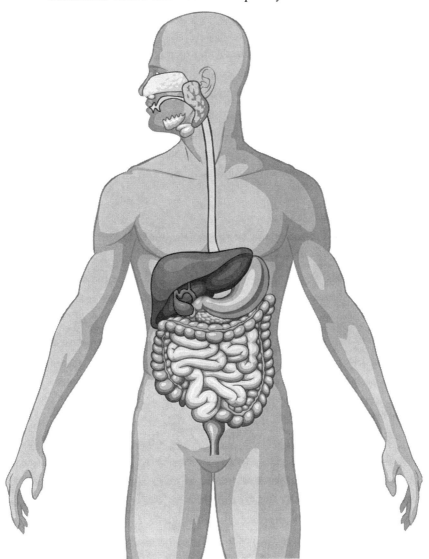

Figure 10. Digestive system. (BigStockPhoto.com © Oguz Aral)

Colon Cancer and Vitamin D

Like many other cancers, the risk of developing colon cancer relates to vitamin D blood levels. Adequate exposure to sunshine can actually prevent one from developing colon cancer, one of the most common cancers from which people suffer. While the fact that the sun can prevent colon cancer from developing may sound questionable to some, there is a lot of science to back this statement up.

In 1985, the prestigious medical journal, *The Lancet*, published an article by Dr. Cedric Garland that showed that those with the lowest vitamin D and calcium intake had higher rates of colon cancer when compared to those with the highest intake of vitamin D and calcium. Researchers evaluated 1,954 men who completed in-depth health questionnaires that covered 28 days of their dietary habits. The researchers took into account smoking, BMI, alcohol consumption, and fat intake into their formulas, and the results were:

> Those people who consumed the least vitamin D and calcium had a one in twenty-five risk of developing colon cancer while those who took the most vitamin D and calcium had a one in seventy-one chance of developing colon cancer, almost three times less risk.

This study, in addition to the Garland 1980 study, started an avalanche of studies that would further investigate the relationship between sunlight, vitamin D, calcium, and colon cancer. However, many healthcare professionals questioned the significance of the data.

A 1993 study by Roberd M. Bostick, MD, MPH (Department of Family Practice and Community Health, Medical School, University of Minnesota Minneapolis, MN), set out to answer whether high levels of calcium, vitamin D, and dairy intake could really protect against colon cancer. The results showed that both calcium and vitamin D decreased the risk of colon cancer, by 48% and 46%, respectively, although the findings were questioned because scientists claimed the results did not reach statistical significance.

A 1998 review by Dr. María Elena Martinez (Arizona Cancer Center, University of Arizona Health Sciences Center) of 20 small scientific studies of vitamin D and colon cancer yielded inconclusive results. She summarized, "The available results for vitamin D suggest that this micronutrient is inversely associated with risk, but, given the scarcity of data additional studies are needed to investigate this relation in more detail."

Fortunately, as time passed, leading vitamin D researchers conducted a number of quality studies. These studies and their findings helped catapult vitamin D's relation to colon cancer into the mainstream.

In a 2002 study, Dr. Michael Freedman (National Cancer Institute, Maryland) evaluated breast and colon cancer rates in the U.S. The study reviewed cancer deaths from 1984 to 1995 in 24 states. The researchers compared those who died from cancer to those who died from other causes. They then evaluated age, sex, race, socioeconomic status, physical activity, and job exposure to sunlight. Interestingly, Dr. Freedman found that those who lived in sunnier areas or had jobs with more sunlight exposure were 17% less likely to die from colon cancer, independent of their physical activity levels. In essence, this study showed 17% less cancer in those who had more sunshine exposure.

> **"Low levels of vitamin D may be associated with increased cancer incidence and mortality in men, particularly for digestive system cancers."**

Other studies have supported the correlation between levels of the sunshine vitamin and the risk of developing colon cancer. In 2006, Edward Giovannucci, MD, ScD (Harvard School of Public Health), and colleagues published a study in the *Journal of the National Cancer Institute*, reporting on cancer among 47,800 men from the years 1986 to 2000. Within this group, they documented 4,286 cases of total cancers and 2,025 deaths from these cancers. Further analysis of the data by the researchers showed that, for every increase of 10 ng/ml (25 nmol/L) of vitamin D in the blood, there was a 17% reduction in total cancer incidence, a 29% reduction in total cancer deaths, and a whopping 37% reduction in colon cancer incidence. Giovannucci concluded that, "Low levels of vitamin D may be associated with increased cancer incidence and mortality in men, particularly for digestive system cancers."

The researchers went on to state that an additional 1,500 IU of vitamin D were required each day to raise one's blood by 10 ng/ml (25 nmol/L). Since blood levels of 50 ng/ml (125 nmol/L) are optimal, one would need to take the equivalent of 7,500 IU daily of vitamin D, less if one has adequate sunlight exposure.

Another study, published in 2004, showed similar benefits of vitamin D on colon cancer. Diane Feskanich, ScD (Assistant Professor at the Department of Medicine, Brigham & Women's Hospital and Harvard Medical School), and her colleagues identified 193 colon cancer cases in women 46 to 78 years of age. Two control patients without cancer were matched for each person with cancer. Among people with the highest level of vitamin D, a 47% decrease in distal colon cancer was present when compared to those with the lowest vitamin D blood levels. The authors went on to conclude:

From these results and supporting evidence from previous studies, we conclude that higher plasma levels of vitamin D 25-OH are associated with a lower risk of colorectal cancer in older women, particularly for cancers at the distal colon and rectum.

> ## "The results showed that those with more vitamin D in their blood could decrease colon cancer risk by 50%"

A study by Edward D. Gorham, MPH, PhD (Naval Health Research Center, University of California San Diego, School of Medicine) evaluated people who took 1,000 IU daily of vitamin D and achieved vitamin D blood levels greater than 33 ng/ml (82.5 nmol/L). They were compared to those with vitamin D blood levels under 13 ng/ml (32.5 nmol/L), a group that took less than 100 IU of vitamin D a day. The results showed that those with more vitamin D in their blood could decrease colon cancer risk by 50%. This is amazing, especially for the number 3 cancer killer in the U.S. Do you know what your vitamin D level is?

Another study by Joan M. Lappe, PhD (Osteoporosis Research Center, Creighton University, Omaha) concluded, "Improving calcium and vitamin D nutritional status substantially reduces all cancer risk in post-menopausal women," to the tune of almost 60%.

As if the above studies are not convincing enough, here is another. Dr. Gorham and colleagues conducted a meta-analysis in 2007, reviewing five studies that included 535 cases of colon cancer. The results showed that those who had serum blood levels of vitamin D greater than 33 ng/ml (82.5 nmol/L) also had 50% less colon cancer when compared to those with vitamin D blood levels under 12 ng/ml (30 nmol/L). These findings were consistent with Dr. Edward Gorham's prior study, which showed a similar reduction. The 2007 study went on to conclude, "The evidence to date suggests that daily intake of 1,000 to 2,000 IU/day of vitamin D3 could reduce the incidence of colorectal with minimal risk." A 50% reduction in colon cancer is an amazing result! There is not one drug on the market that can achieve anything close to that.

In all fairness, not all studies showed protection from vitamin D. One study by Jean Wactawski-Wende, PhD (University of Buffalo), and colleagues, published in the *New England Journal of Medicine,* showed no relationship between vitamin D supplementation and cancer protection after following patients for 7 years. However, in that study, people took only 400 IU of vitamin D. Such a small dose is unlikely to show much benefit. In addition, vitamin D blood levels went unmeasured in that study, so there was no way to know if any vitamin D deficiencies, if present, were adequately treated.

Based on the results from prior studies and from my personal experience, 400 IU of vitamin D does not make much of a difference in blood levels of vitamin D. However, this study is important, as it shows the current recommendations are too low to have any significant benefit on cancer prevention. The daily minimum needs to be raised to at least 2,000 IU of vitamin D. If you are relying on a multivitamin to give your body sufficient vitamin D to prevent anything but rickets, you will not get enough.

Dr. Madrid, I Already Have Colon Cancer, What Can I Do?

What if you or a family member has received a diagnosis of colon cancer? Is it too late to benefit from vitamin D? I have good news for you! Vitamin D supplementation can still be of benefit.

Mr. Rodriguez (name changed), a patient of mine, was diagnosed with colon cancer. One year earlier, he had a colonoscopy that showed he had a precancerous colon polyp. The colon specialist referred him to a surgeon, who recommended he have part of his colon removed. The patient thought this was too drastic a move and decided to wait and see what happened. I told him that my recommendation was the same as the surgeon.

At the time, I was not aware of the evidence of vitamin D preventing colon cancer. Six months later, Mr. Rodriguez returned to my office with complaints of rectal bleeding with his bowel movements. I referred him back to the colon specialist who subsequently sent him to the surgeon after a colonoscopy showed the polyp had developed into cancer. When the surgeon took Mr. Rodriguez to the operating room, he encountered a tumor too big for surgery. The surgeon closed up the incision and referred Mr. Rodriguez to an oncologist for radiation and chemotherapy, in hopes of shrinking the tumor to enable surgery. By this time, I had become aware of vitamin D's anti-cancer benefits. I checked Mr. Rodriguez' level. Curiously, his level was 12 ng/ml (30 nmol/L), very deficient. I began immediate treatment with vitamin D supplementation. Eventually, Mr. Rodriguez had his surgery, while continuing his vitamin D supplementation. To this day, he is alive and I expect him to do well. I am not claiming vitamin D was the answer, but when taken in conjunction with the best treatments his cancer doctor had to offer, Mr. Rodriguez was given another chance at life.

As reported in the breast cancer section of this book, a study conducted in Norway by Dr. Trude Robsahm, MSc (Senior researcher at The Cancer Registry of Norway) showed that those diagnosed with colon cancer during the summer and fall, when vitamin D blood levels are higher, had better prognoses than those diagnosed in the winter and spring, when levels are lowest.

Similar findings exist for lung cancer, breast cancer, and prostate cancer.

A 2008 study by Kimmie Ng, MD, MPH (Dana-Farber Cancer Institute, Boston), and colleagues was published in the *Journal of Clinical Oncology*. In the study, researchers measured the vitamin D levels of 304 colon cancer patients. The results showed that those with vitamin D blood levels above 40 ng/ml (100 nmol/L) were 48% less likely *to die* when compared to those with levels less than 16.6 ng/ml (41.5 nmol/L). This study demonstrates that it is never too late to start supplementing your diet with vitamin D and increasing your sunshine exposure.

In other words if you, or a loved one, have been diagnosed with colon cancer—or any other cancer for that matter—you need to immediately begin vitamin D supplementation. It is important that you ask your doctor to check your vitamin D blood level in order to make sure you take a dose that will optimize your blood to levels above 50 ng/ml (125 nmol/L). When a person has cancer, calcium levels need to be monitored, as increased vitamin D supplementation can result in even higher blood calcium levels that sometimes are associated with cancers. In addition, if you have cancer, consider giving your physician a copy of this book—especially your surgeon and cancer specialist (oncologist).

> **Those diagnosed with colon cancer during the summer and fall seasons, when vitamin D blood levels are higher, had better prognosis than those diagnosed in the winter and spring, when vitamin D levels are lower.**

In summary, the research shows that vitamin D and increased sunlight exposure help prevent colon cancer from beginning. In addition, higher vitamin D blood levels can also help improve survival for those already diagnosed with colon cancer. The evidence is clear, vitamin D has anticancer properties. I recommend taking at least 2,000 IU /daily. However, it is important to have routine blood level tests to make sure the dosages being taken are enough to get vitamin D levels above 50 ng/ml (125 nmol/L).

Prostate Health and Men

The prostate is a gland positioned between the bladder and the colon in men. The word prostate, is Greek in origin, originally, prostátēs, defined as "one standing before" or "protector". The main function of the prostate is to secrete a clear, alkaline fluid to help transport sperm during ejaculation. The alkalinity helps to neutralize the acidity of the female vagina, protecting the male sperm and allowing fertilization to occur. The prostate can become infected, a condition called *prostatitis*. When the prostate is enlarged, it is referred to as benign prostatic hyperplasia (BPH). When the prostate has the presence of cancer cells, the man has prostate cancer.

Benign Prostate Hyperplasia (BPH)

When the prostate enlarges, a man will find himself having difficulty urinating. Most men with BPH awake 1 to 5 times a night just to urinate. In addition, they might notice difficulty initiating urination and will have dribbling of urine upon completion. The simple fact of arising multiple times during the night can obviously make getting a good night's sleep difficult. Fortunately, there are several things a man can do to minimize the swelling of the prostate so he and his partner can have a restful night.

From a lifestyle perspective, eating healthy foods such as whole grains and organic fruits and vegetables is beneficial. Some experts, including myself, recommend avoiding caffeine and alcohol, or at least keeping it to a bare minimum. Many patients have benefited from taking the herbal supplement, saw palmetto, at a minimum dose of 320 mg daily. When a man comes to my office complaining of symptoms of an enlarged prostate, I usually recommend that he start off with these changes to see if they benefit. Many patients benefit, but not all.

When these interventions don't work, there are medicines that doctors can prescribe to help shrink the prostate. Fortunately, these medicines work quite well for the majority who take them. Like all medicines, side effects can cause some to discontinue their use.

For those who still have difficulty in spite of trying various strategies, surgical intervention can be an option. However, side effects of surgery can result in urinary incontinence or permanent impotence. As common as BPH is, the good news is that there is no evidence that it puts a man at increased risk for developing prostate cancer.

Prostate Cancer

Cancer of the prostate affects 1 in 6 men and causes 10% of all cancer deaths. Prostate cancer is so common, that an estimated 90% of men over age 90 show evidence of microscopic prostate cancer. However, it is unlikely to be a cause of death for men in this age group, as heart disease and dying of natural causes are more likely to occur before death from prostate cancer.

Ask any man over 40 how a prostate exam is done and he will tell you, usually with apprehension, a fearful look, or with a smirk on his face. While a blood test for a prostate-specific antigen (PSA) is commonly ordered, the physician's gloved index finger is the best way to identify those at risk for prostate cancer. If a nodule or abnormality is felt, the physician may recommend a prostate biopsy to rule out the presence of cancerous cells.

While this test is not pleasant for the physician and is usually quite uncomfortable for the man, it is an important part of a complete health physical. I tell my patients that 30 seconds of discomfort once a year is definitely a fair trade-off to prevent dying from prostate cancer. Most agree. I had one patient jokingly ask, "Gee, Doc, are you at least going to take me out to dinner and a movie first?" I happily go along with whatever the patient needs to "break the ice."

The doctor will conduct a digital rectal exam with a gloved finger. By doing this, the doctor can feel the prostate gland and detect the presence or absence of prostate abnormalities. It is not uncommon for a man to have a normal PSA blood test while having evidence of prostate cancer on exam. Therefore, men should not rely solely on the blood test.

Because prostate cancer accounts for 10% of all male cancer deaths, diagnosis is essential. While prostate cancer is uncommon before age 55, many experts believe it is important to screen men over age 40. Others recommend screening start at age 50. The younger a man is when diagnosed with prostate cancer, the more aggressive the cancer is. African-American men are at higher risk and, when diagnosed, are usually at more advanced stages of the cancer compared to Caucasians, Asians, and Hispanics. Those men who have diets high in red meat, dairy products, and refined foods are also at higher risk, while those who eat more fruits, vegetables, soy, and green tea have lower risk.

A study by Marilyn Tseng (National Institutes of Health) and colleagues showed those with the highest intake of dairy foods were 2.2 times more likely to develop prostate cancer. A sensible diet in moderation cannot be overstated and should be embraced by all.

Further, if you have a family history of prostate cancer, it is important to take extra precautions to protect your health. Making lifestyle changes now can ultimately prove to be lifesaving. Fortunately, studies have shown that those with higher levels of vitamin D are protected from developing prostate cancer when compared to those with lower blood levels. Do you know what your blood level of vitamin D is? If you are a woman, what is your husband or father's vitamin D level? Asking them to get it checked can save their lives.

Risk factors for prostate cancer

- Age over 50
- Race—African-American
- Diets high in fat and dairy products
- Metabolic syndrome
- Sedentary lifestyle
- Family history
- Vitamin D deficiency

Studies have shown that those with prostate cancer are more likely to be vitamin D deficient than those without prostate cancer. Fortunately, supplementation is inexpensive. It is definitely more cost efficient to prevent disease than to treat it once it has started.

Being overweight, obese or having metabolic syndrome (diagnosed if you have any three: (1) high blood sugar or diabetes, (2) high blood pressure, (3) overweight, (4) low HDL cholesterol, or (5) elevated triglycerides) is believed to be a risk factor for many cancers, including prostate cancer. Having metabolic syndrome is an indication of poor diet and lack of exercise. However, a recent study explains a possible link between metabolic syndrome and prostate cancer.

Pentti Tuohimaa, MD, PhD (University of Tampere Medical School and Department of Clinical Chemistry, Finland) and colleagues conducted a study on 132 prostate cancer patients and 456 men without prostate cancer. The patients came from a group of 18,939 Finnish middle-aged men. The results are showed in Table 10 and show how various risk factors influence the risk of developing prostate cancer when compared to a person with a BMI <28, no high blood pressure, good (HDL) cholesterol above 40, and a vitamin D level above 16 ng/ml (40nmol/L).

Table 10. Effect of health factors on risk of prostate cancer

Over-weight (BMI >28)	High Blood Pressure	Low good (HDL <40) cholesterol	Vitamin D level <16 ng/ml (40nmol/L)	Risk of Prostate Cancer
X				37% increased risk
X	X			53% increased risk
X	X	X		236% increased risk
X	X	X	X	703% increased risk

This led the authors to conclude that the prostate cancer risk associated with metabolic syndrome is strongly conditioned by levels of vitamin D in the blood. In other words, a poor diet and lack of exercise, in addition to vitamin D deficiency, significantly increase the risk of developing prostate cancer.

Aruna V. Krishnan, PhD (Department of Endocrinology, Stanford University School of Medicine, California), and colleagues studied vitamin D. Their study suggested that vitamin D inhibits prostaglandins, the inflammatory chemicals that, when present in high levels, increase the risk of prostate cancer. The authors went on to conclude that vitamin D regulates numerous pathways that function in the prevention of prostate cancer. In essence, in the absence of adequate vitamin D, prostate cancer is allowed to grow and spread throughout the body.

Larisa Nonn, PhD (Department of Urology, Stanford University School of Medicine, California), and other researchers published a study in 2006 in which they conclude that vitamin D decreases the amount of prostate inflammation and, therefore, prevents prostate cancer through various biochemical pathways. This important study provides a possible reason vitamin D can help prevent prostate cancer.

> **"The study went on to show that those with higher levels of vitamin D were 60% to 70% less likely to develop total and aggressive prostate cancer"**

Haojie Li, MD, PhD (Department of Medicine, Brigham and Women's Hospital & Harvard School of Medicine), and colleagues published a study in 2007 that involved 14,916 male patients who were followed for 18 years. All these men were without diagnosed prostate cancer at the time they entered the study. The study went on to show that those with higher levels of vitamin D were 60% to 70% less likely to develop total and aggressive prostate cancer. The authors concluded that a large proportion of U.S. men had suboptimal vitamin D levels and that vitamin D could play an important role in prostate cancer prevention. I could not agree more! All men need to have their vitamin D levels checked.

Genetics of Prostate Cancer

While genetics and family history strongly influence one's medical future, they do not determine one's destiny. It is important that you do not allow yourself to fall victim to your "genetic profile". Over the next decade, people will be able to order tests to see whether or not they are at risk for certain diseases and cancers, including prostate cancer. While that information can be both helpful and scary, it does not imply one's fate. Personal choices we make every day about our diet and exercise routine can alter our genetic futures for the better.

A study in 1997 on the genetics of vitamin D showed that certain people with prostate cancer could actually have defective vitamin D receptor genes (VDRs), which prevent them from realizing the preventive benefits of vitamin D. This was an exciting study and the results were promising.

However, a meta-analysis published in 2003 reviewed 14 studies on the genetics of VDRs and prostate cancer. The study concluded that the four polymorphisms (VDRs) are unlikely to be major determinants of susceptibility to prostate cancer on a wide population basis.

A more recent study by Esther M. John, PhD (Northern California Cancer Center), published in 2005, on the genetics of prostate cancer, concluded, "Our findings support the hypothesis that sun exposure and VDR polymorphisms together play an important role in the etiology (cause) of prostate cancer."

So what is the answer to these two seemingly contradictory findings? Do vitamin D receptors influence prostate cancer or not? Well, the jury is not yet in. This is a growing area of research and, in the future, certain genetic testing will allow us to identify those at higher risk for developing prostate cancer. It is plausible that, if there is a group of men who are unable to recognize vitamin D molecules in their entirety, perhaps this group can take vitamin D analogues or possibly extremely high doses of vitamin D than would normally be used in the general population.

In a follow-up editorial, Sue Ann Ingles, DrPhH (Department of Preventive Medicine, University of Southern California), commented in a 2007 paper that the studies of the genetics of vitamin VDRs have been inconsistent. However, she went on to state that most of these studies did not take into consideration the blood levels of vitamin D. As shown, this is where the evidence lies for cancer prevention. Studies show higher vitamin D blood levels are associated with lower cancer risk.

I think the next decade will help elucidate the genetics of VDRs and the cancer risk some gene variations can pose. However, one thing appears clear—optimizing one's vitamin D levels, either through adequate sunshine exposure and/or sufficient vitamin D supplementation, can help decrease the odds of developing prostate cancer in men. We can safely do this with no lasting side effects. This is an ongoing field of scientific research; the potential epidemiological benefits are enormous.

Cervical Cancer

The cervix connects the uterus to the vagina. In Latin, cervix means *neck*. Every time a woman goes for her yearly Pap smear, she is screened for cervical cancer. Samples of cells are taken from the cervix, and a pathologist will review the cells to search for the presence of abnormal cells, which may indicate pre-cancer or cancer.

While cervical cancer is a leading killer of women around the world, it has become a rare cancer in the U.S. This is due, in large part, to the mass screening of women with the Pap smear exam. With screening for cervical cancer, physicians are now able to treat patients who are in the precancerous stage. A majority of the women who still die in the USA from cervical cancer do so because they did not have routine Pap smears.

Cervical cancer is the number 10 cancer in the U.S., affects 9,000 to 12,000 women, and kills about 4,000 women annually. Worldwide, cervical cancer is more dangerous and is the fifth-most common cancer, annually affecting almost 500,000 women, and killing about 270,000 women. In less-developed countries, cervical cancer is the second-leading cause of cancer deaths.

Risk factors for cervical cancer include the following:

- Infection with human papillomavirus
- Chlamydia infection
- Diets low in fruits and vegetables
- Smoking
- Immune suppression
- Multiple sexual partners
- Birth control pills
- Multiple pregnancies
- Lower socio-economic status
- Family history

Evidence shows that the presence of human papillomavirus, or HPV, increases a woman's risk for developing cervical cancer. Fortunately, most women who are exposed to this virus will clear it from their body through their body's natural defense mechanisms. In fact, an estimated 99% of women who test positive for HPV will eventually test negative.

However, the 1% who don't clear the virus are at increased risk for cervical cancer. Women who smoke and have multiple sexual partners, especially at a young age, are at increased risk for developing cervical cancer.

Maintaining a healthy immune system is vital in preventing HPV from over-taking the cervix and transforming into cancer. In underdeveloped countries where food, hygiene, and nutrition are lacking, a weaker immune system is more likely to occur.

In recent years, pharmaceutical giant Merck, began to market their anti-HPV vaccine. The hope was that mass vaccination could eliminate cervical cancer in the U.S. and in other developed countries that could afford the vaccine.

Merck's Gardasil.com web site explains:

GARDASIL is the only cervical cancer vaccine that helps protect against 4 types of human papillomavirus (HPV): 2 types that cause 70% of cervical cancer cases, and 2 more types that cause 90% of genital warts cases. GARDASIL is for girls and young women ages 9 to 26.

Experts hope the number of cervical cancer deaths in the U.S. and Europe will significantly decrease over the next 20 to 25 years from the vaccine. While cervical cancer is a horrible disease, it affects so few that this vaccine can make only a small dent in the overall cancer mortality rate. According to the *National PBM Drug Monograph*, it is estimated that for each 67 women who have the vaccine series, 1 low grade, abnormal pap smear will be prevented. Further, 250 women will need to receive the vaccine series in order to prevent a high grade abnormal Pap smear or cervical cancer. The vaccine has become controversial; the FDA reports over 20 cases of death among young girls after taking the vaccine, although causation has not been established.

Proposed legislation in various states to make this vaccine mandatory among young girls has met challenges. During the later part of 2008, Merck was successful in persuading the government to require Gardasil for all immigrant women coming into the U.S. The attempt to legislate vaccination of young girls has become a controversial issue within many circles, as no vaccines are truly mandatory, only recommended. While preventing cancer is important, many experts still question the effectiveness of Gardasil.

Dr. Diane Harper, co-inventor of the vaccine, had this to say about Gardasil, as reported on the Alliance for Human Research Protection website:

> Giving it to 11-year olds is a great big public health experiment… This vaccine should not be mandated for 11-year old girls…It's not been tested in little girls for efficacy. At 11, these girls don't get cervical cancer—they won't know for 25 years if they will get cervical cancer.

Many are concerned that the co-inventor of the vaccine is not entirely on board with the current recommendations about the vaccine's administration. Dr. Harper went on to comment that she was concerned that those who get the vaccine would believe that they were protected from cervical cancer and not have their Pap smears. This will put these women at risk of dying from cervical cancer. It is important that all physicians who recommend the Gardasil vaccine to their young patients remind them that a yearly Pap smear is still vital in helping prevent cervical cancer.

The cost of the three-shot series and the administration of it is about $600. The Merck gardasil.com web site further states: "The side effects include pain, swelling, itching, and redness at the injection site, fever, nausea, dizziness, vomiting, and fainting. GARDASIL is given as 3 injections over 6 months."

While there are not many studies on vitamin D and cervical cancer, one by Dr. Michael Friedrich (Department of Gynecology and Obstetrics, University of Saarland, Homburg/Saar, Germany) suggested that cervical cancer is minimized by optimizing vitamin D levels. If proven effective, the cost-benefit analysis would show that massive vitamin D supplementation and increased fortification of food products would be far more beneficial to our national health and provide far more cancer protection than vaccination with Gardasil. The combination of the two interventions may be even more effective.

Studies have shown that vitamin D can be of benefit to those with early signs of cervical cancer. A study by Dr. Michael Friedrich and colleagues reported:

...25(OH)D3-1-alpha-hydroxylase is expressed in normal cervical tissue, in cervical cancer...cells. Thus, normal cervical and cervical cancer cells seem to be able to synthesize 1-alpha, 25(OH)2D3 that may be of significant importance for the growth control in normal and malignant cervical tissue. Normal cervical tissue and cervical cancer cells may be new targets for cancer prevention or cancer treatment with precursors of biologically active vitamin D analogues.

In other words, the cells of the cervix have the enzyme necessary to use vitamin D, and this could help prevent cervical cancer. This is the same enzyme present in breast tissue and the colon, which allows vitamin D to prevent cancer.

This area of cancer research is a growing field and there are not many other studies to support the correlation between vitamin D and cervical cancer at this time. However, I am certain that over the next several years, studies will show whether vitamin D is of any benefit in cervical cancer prevention and treatment. In the meantime, it is important that women speak with their family doctor or ob-gyn about routine Pap smears. Also, discuss with your physician if Gardasil vaccination is right for you or your daughters.

Ovarian Cancer

The ovaries are amazing organs and are part of the female reproductive system. They are responsible for producing mature eggs each month that will be receptive for fertilization, should it occur. The ovaries are about the size of small grapes. The word ovary comes from the Latin, *uva,* meaning grape.

When a baby girl is born, she is equipped with about 1,000,000 follicles, each of which has an opportunity to become a mature egg. By the time she begins puberty, they number about 400,000 follicles. During each month, about 15 to 25 follicles will begin maturation, and one will become a mature egg. The body will absorb the rest. In addition to producing eggs, the ovaries are also responsible for estrogen creation. When a woman reaches menopause, the ovaries stop producing estrogen. Unfortunately, it is at this time when ovarian cancer is most likely to occur.

Ovarian cancer is one of the more difficult cancers to screen. While there has been much talk about the CA-125 blood test, experts are split as to whether this test is of any value. Not everyone with ovarian cancer will have an elevated level and not everyone who has an elevated level has ovarian cancer.

Risk factors for ovarian cancer include the following:

- Obesity
- Age > 50
- Not having children
- Hormone replacement therapy
- Personal history of breast cancer
- Poor diet

While cancer of the ovaries occurs less frequently than breast and colon cancers, it still affects 1 in 71 women and accounts for 6% of all cancer deaths. About 26,000 women are diagnosed with the cancer each year, and 14,500 women will die from it. Women with a family history of ovarian cancer are at increased risk and vitamin D deficiency also appears to be a risk factor, as it is for many other cancers.

Women with ovarian cancer are usually over 50 years of age at the time of diagnosis and may present with pain in the lower abdomen and feeling bloated. Ovarian cancer is best detected by a pelvic ultrasound or CT exam of the pelvis; however, physicians also perform a bimanual exam of the ovaries during a Pap exam in an attempt to palpate enlarged ovaries.

> **"Women aged 45 to 54 had 5 times more ovarian cancer if they lived in the northern states, where there was less sunlight, than if they lived in the southern states"**

A 1994 study published in the *International Journal of Epidemiology* by Dr. Ellen Lefkowitz and Dr. Cedric Garland of UC San Diego showed that sunlight exposure could protect against ovarian cancer. In their study, they showed that women aged 45 to 54 had 5 times more ovarian cancer if they lived in the northern states, where there was less sunlight, than if they lived in the southern states.

A separate study by Dr. Eduardo Salazar-Martinez (Center for Research in Population Health, National Institute of Public Health, Cuernavaca, Morelos, Mexico) and colleagues conducted in Mexico also showed a relationship between vitamin D intake and ovarian cancer. Researchers concluded:

> The diet of the Mexican population is rich in carbohydrates; in Mexico corn intake is the main energy source. On the other hand, vitamins such as retinol and vitamin D were shown to be associated with this neoplasm (ovarian cancer) in a protective way; nevertheless, further studies are necessary to allow us to corroborate our results. This is the first attempt in our country that relates the Mexican diet to ovarian cancer.

In other words, those who reported a higher intake of vitamin D had less ovarian cancer. Like cervical cancer studies, ovarian cancer studies are limited. Part of the problem is the fact that ovarian cancer is not as prevalent as breast and colon cancer; therefore, studies of less common cancers are hard to come by. However, over time I expect more research to give us a clearer picture of the relationship between vitamin D and ovarian cancer. In the meantime, it is vital that women see their physicians for their yearly physical exams. In addition, it is important that women optimize their vitamin D levels due to the enormous overall health benefits associated with levels above 50 ng/ml (125 nmol/L).

Pancreatic Cancer

Cancer of the pancreas is the fourth-leading cause of cancer deaths in the U.S. Risk factors for pancreatic cancer include older age, smoking, diabetes and low vitamin D intake, to name a few. Unfortunately, it is also one of the most deadly cancers and has an overall low survival rate. Since prevention is always the key, preventing pancreatic cancer is vital; treatment options are limited. However, even prevention is a challenge. According to the American Cancer Society, 38,000 people are diagnosed with this cancer yearly and 34,000 people die. Only 5% of people diagnosed with pancreatic cancer will be alive at 5 years. This is truly a serious cancer with few who survive. The risk factors for pancreatic cancer include:

- Older age
- Race (African-Americans more likely to get it than Caucasians)
- Smoking
- High fat and meat diet
- Diabetes
- Environmental exposure to gasoline and pesticide
- Low vitamin D intake

In a 2006 study by Halcyon Skinner, PhD, MPH (Department of Preventive Medicine, Feinberg School of Medicine, Northwestern University, Chicago, Illinois), a preventive effect of vitamin D against pancreatic cancer was seen. In a prospective study, Dr. Skinner and colleagues evaluated 46,771 men ages 40-75 years of age as of 1986 and 75,427 women ages 38 to 65 years as of 1984 (the Nurses' Health Study). The results showed that those who consumed more than 600 IU of vitamin D daily compared to those who consumed less than 150 IU daily had a 41% decreased risk of pancreatic cancer.

> **"Those with higher vitamin D levels had 51% less pancreatic cancer than those with the lowest blood levels of vitamin D"**

In addition, a 2006 study by Edward Giovannucci, MD, ScD (Harvard School of Public Health), published in the *Journal of the National Institute*, showed that those with higher vitamin D levels had 51% less pancreatic cancer than those with the lowest blood levels of vitamin D.

African-Americans typically have lower levels of vitamin D than Caucasians, which could explain why they are at greater risk for pancreatic cancer. The studies that support the vitamin D and pancreatic cancer hypothesis are still sparse and over time, more research will help delineate the relationship. However, in my opinion, vitamin D blood levels will likely prove to be a strong risk factor for pancreatic cancer prevention. Further, smoking cessation, a healthy diet, and blood sugar control can help prevent pancreatic cancer. The take home message here is that you need to have your vitamin D level checked. I recommend a goal of >50 ng/ml (125 nmol/L) for overall health.

Melanoma Skin Cancer

Melanoma is the most dreaded of all skin cancers. It will affect 1 in 41 men and 1 in 62 women in the U.S. alone. According to the National Cancer Institute, 62,480 people will be diagnosed with melanoma in the U.S. in 2008; 8,420 will die. Worldwide, 160,000 people will be diagnosed; 48,000 will die. While only accounting for 5% of all skin cancers, it is the most dangerous. There are certain characteristics that make a skin lesion suspicious for melanoma. Many use *ABCDE* of melanoma to help identify the risk associated.

A = asymmetry of the lesion, that is one half is different than the other

B= borders are irregularly shaped

C= color is dark but may have variations of brown, black and tan

D= diameter is bigger than a pencil eraser (6 mm)

E= evolving lesion over time

Nonmelanoma skin cancers, specifically, basal cell carcinoma and squamous cell carcinoma, account for the other 95% of skin cancers and are not generally life-threatening. They simply cause local tissue destruction so should be excised when present.

Melanin is the substance in our skin that gives us pigment. Specific cells called melanocytes make melanin. Everyone has melanocytes that are capable of producing melanin to one degree or another. Melanocytes have receptors for vitamin D. In other words, vitamin D affects regulation of melanocyte genes. The darker our skin, the more melanin we have; the lighter our skin, the less melanin we have. Scientists have discovered the genes that cause some people to have more melanin than others. These genes represent only a small portion of tens of thousands of human genes we have in common. In fact, it is estimated that humans have 99.98% of our DNA in common, whereas .02% accounts for the differences we see when we look at each other.

Scientists postulate that when early humans migrated out of Africa and the Middle East to Northern Europe and Asia, the mutation that resulted in lighter skin allowed vitamin D production in areas where the sun does not shine much. This mutation was necessary for human survival and calcium absorption.

Like any cell in our body, melanocytes have control mechanisms that keep their growth in balance. When a cell loses its ability to control its division, growth becomes erratic and cancerous melanoma results.

Albinos, however, have a genetic defect that results in an absence of melanin. Contrary to popular belief, however, even albinos are susceptible to melanoma skin cancer. They can get amelanocytic melanoma, according to John J. Di Giovanna, MD, a dermatologist at the National Cancer Institute.

Most assume that excess sunlight causes melanoma, but this is only part of the story. The American Cancer Society even states on their website that "We do not yet know exactly what causes melanoma skin cancer. But we do know that certain risk factors are linked to this disease."

UV light from the sun is definitely a risk factor. However, those with light skin are more susceptible to the negative effects that excess ultraviolet light has to offer.

Jim Shaffer Jr. (real name) was a sun worshiper. In the 1980s, he spent an enormous amount of time in sun-soaked Southern California. His work required him to spend a lot time in the sun, and when he was not working, he would spend his weekends jet skiing and boating on the Colorado River. Sunscreen use was the exception, and not the rule. In 2001, Jim was diagnosed with melanoma on the forehead. Fortunately, surgeons at Cedars-Sinai were able to remove it. Immediately thereafter, the sun became the enemy to both him and his wife. Sunscreen use became the norm.

Over the next 3 years, Jim developed two other sites of melanoma, even though he now avoided unprotected sun exposure. Jim had no family history of melanoma. Surely his melanoma must have been caused by his sun exposure, correct? As obvious as this assertion may seem, some health care professionals actually challenge this. Believe it or not, the question of whether sun exposure primarily causes melanoma is still a controversy in many professional circles. There are other risk factors also, these include:

- Sun exposure that resulted in blistering sun burns prior to age twenty
- Family history of melanoma
- Large number of moles on the body
- Red-haired and fair-skinned individuals face increased risk
- Older age
- Poor Diet
- Weak immune system

Johan Moan, PhD (Institute for Cancer Research, Montebello Institute of Physics, University of Oslo, Norway), cited studies in his paper that showed melanoma is more common among people who work indoors rather than outdoors. Also, there are more melanomas that arise on areas that get less sun exposure, such as the trunk and legs. Some even get melanoma on the bottoms of their feet—a form of cancer called acral melanoma.

This is the opposite of what most have been taught, including physicians. However, Dr. Johan Moan commented that he believes a large number of melanomas are related to sun exposure. But apparently, sunshine is only part of the cause.

However, not everyone agrees that more sun always results in more skin melanoma. Some have even suggested that sunscreen use actually promotes more melanoma. In 1992, Cedric F. Garland, DrPH (Moores Cancer Center University of California, San Diego), stated:

It is time to review the efficacy of sunscreens in the prevention of melanoma and basal cell carcinomas. Untested but widespread public health recommendations concerning the use of sunscreens for the prevention of skin cancer maybe more harmful than advice to control sun exposure by more traditional means.

He basically said the use of sunscreens for the prevention of skin cancer may be more harmful. Why would this be? Does sunscreen promote melanoma skin cancer? A study in 2000 by Johan Westerdahl, PhD (Department of Surgery, University Hospital, Lund, Sweden) actually suggested that sunscreen use could increase risk of melanoma, as people tend to stay in the sun longer than they would otherwise. This increased exposure to UV light increases DNA mutations, thereby promoting cancer.

A study published in 2003 by Leslie Dennis, MS, PhD (Department of Epidemiology, College of Public Health, University of Iowa, Iowa), did not see evidence that sunscreen caused melanoma. She concluded:

No association was seen between melanoma and sunscreen use. Failure to control for confounding factors may explain previous reports of positive associations linking melanoma to sunscreen use. In addition, it may take decades to detect a protective association between melanoma and use of the newer formulations of sunscreens.

So what is the answer? If excess sun exposure causes melanoma, why do most melanomas occur more on non-sun exposed areas? If sunscreen is supposed to protect us from melanoma, why would some studies suggest it may promote melanoma?

According to researcher Harri Vainio (International Agency for Research on Cancer, Lyon Cedex, France)

No conclusion could be drawn about the cancer-preventive activity of topical sunscreens against basal-cell carcinoma and cutaneous melanoma. The use of sunscreens can extend the duration of intentional sun exposure, such as sunbathing. Such an extension may increase the risk for cutaneous melanoma. The workshop warned against relying solely on sunscreens for protection from ultraviolet radiation.

It appears that there is no clear answer. However, minimizing the risk factors, when at all possible, is a good place to start. Ensuring that one does not spend too much time in the sun is probably a good idea since UVA light has the ability to cause DNA damage, which can ultimately cause cancer. Make sure your sunscreen protects against both UV-A and UV-B light.

Vitamin D Protects against Melanoma

While the studies that support higher levels of vitamin D and melanoma prevention are minimal, they are at least consistent with the studies of vitamin D and cancer prevention overall. A study by Dr. Peter E. Hutchinson (Departments of Dermatology and Plastic Surgery Leicester Royal Infirmary, Leicester, UK) showed that people who have abnormal VDRs (vitamin D receptors) and are, therefore, unable to utilize vitamin D fully, lose the protective effect against malignant melanoma. The melanocytes (melanin producing cells) essentially become cancerous in the absence of vitamin D.

A laboratory study conducted by Kay W. Colston, PhD (Department of Clinical Biochemistry, St Georges Hospital Medical School London), showed that cell lines of melanoma grew more slowly when exposed to extra vitamin D. In other words, vitamin D prevented cancer cells from growing fast and multiplying.

A 2005 study by Marianne Berwick, PhD, MPH (University of New Mexico, New Mexico Cancer Research Facility), concluded, "Sun exposure is associated with increased survival from melanoma." On the surface, this would appear to be counterintuitive. However, it appears that vitamin D can help control melanin cells if they become cancerous, thereby improving survival once a melanoma is diagnosed. In this situation, supplementing with vitamin D would be more prudent than attempting to get vitamin D from the sun. More studies are needed to further elucidate the beneficial effects of vitamin D and melanoma prevention.

In summary, we know that severe sunburns increase the risk of skin cancer. Specifically, UVA and UVB light waves can damage DNA in cells, including melanocytes. Most sunscreens block out over 99% UVB, the less harmful of the two. In addition, UVB is necessary for the skin to formulate Vitamin D. In essence, sunscreen inhibits our body's ability to make vitamin D.

Since most sunscreens do not typically filter out UVA (they are just beginning to), people will spend more time in the sun, increasing risk for skin damage and skin cancer. It is important to take other measures to protect the skin from the harmful effects of UV damage. Avoiding excess sunlight from 10:00 a.m. to 2:00 p.m. is important to minimize UVA damage. However, getting at least 10 to 15 minutes is important in maintaining one's vitamin D level, which ultimately has anticancer properties. Vitamin D supplementation with 2,000 IU minimum of vitamin D is recommended for optimal vitamin D blood levels. Routine measurement of serum vitamin D is essential to ensure normal levels and to prevent hypercalcemia. Many may need to take higher doses.

SECTION VIII:
FUTURE RESEARCH

There are other areas of vitamin D research that are exciting and show a lot of promise for the future. Some studies have shown that vitamin D protects against the following cancers:

- Kidney cancer
- Endometrial cancer
- Non-Hodgkin's lymphoma

These topics will be discussed in a future edition of this book. Furthermore, scientists from the vitamin D council recently commented, at a vitamin D conference in San Diego, that low levels of vitamin D may be associated with autism. When a child is vitamin D deficient, cells become "leakier," allowing environmental toxins to negatively affect the nervous system. As the research on these areas grows, this information will be shared.

SECTION IX:
MAKE THE CHANGE, TREAT YOUR VITAMIN D DEFICIENCY

"Every body continues in its state of rest, or of uniform motion..., unless it is compelled to change that state by forces impressed upon it" Principia Mathematica "Laws of motion" 1687
- Isaac Newton.

The evidence is clear. If you are not currently taking vitamin D supplements and have not had your vitamin D blood level checked, then you are jeopardizing your health and limiting your longevity. Take the information you have learned in this book and share it with your friends, family members, coworkers, and even your physician. Encourage everyone you know to have his or her vitamin D blood level checked.

Important: Make certain to ask your doctor to check vitamin D 25-OH and not vitamin D 1,25 OH.

It is also important to start increasing your exposure to the sun and enjoy the healing properties it has to offer. However, take care to prevent sunburns. Many experts recommend spending at least 10 to 15 minutes in the sun between 10:00 a.m. and 2:00 p.m., before putting sunscreen on. However, care needs to be taken to prevent excessive sun exposure resulting in skin redness or erythema. If you have darker skin pigment, you may need to spend more time in the sun. If you apply sunscreen, make sure it filters both UVA and UVB light waves in order to minimize sun damage and aging of the skin.

In recent years, the availability of vitamin D3 (cholecalciferol) has become more widespread. Unfortunately, it may still be difficult to find it in some community stores. However, studies show that vitamin D3 is three times more effective than vitamin D2 (ergocalciferol).

The amount of vitamin D found in most multivitamins such as Centrum, Centrum Silver, Kirkland, and other leading vitamins is insufficient. Some calcium/vitamin D combination supplements have the less potent vitamin D2 (ergocalciferol) and not the more potent vitamin D3 (cholecalciferol). While most over-the-counter multivitamins contain 400 IU of vitamin D2 or D3, the evidence shows that this dose is ineffective for over 95% of the population. This level will prevent only rickets. As you have seen, I have been recommending at least 2,000 IU of vitamin D throughout the book.

In a 2006 study published in the *American Journal of Clinical Nutrition*, Heike Bischoff-Ferrari, MD, MPH (Department of Rheumatology and Institute of Physical Medicine, University Hospital Zurich), and colleagues showed that 1,000 IU of vitamin D3 given to healthy adults, brought less than 50% of those who took the vitamin D, to a blood level of 30 ng/ml (75 nmol/L).

Dr. Oz often recommends a dose of 1,000 IU of vitamin D to people; however, the evidence shows that is simply not enough for most people. Many vitamin D experts, including myself, recommend a daily dose of 2,000 IU of vitamin D3 (cholecalciferol). This is the minimum amount recommended for a person who has not checked his or her blood levels.

In reality, the dose you take should depend on your blood levels. For this reason, it is important to have a blood test done. I frequently recommend the following guidelines to my patients.

- If your vitamin D blood level is less than 15 ng/ml (37.5 nmol/L) and you have a normal calcium level, I recommend you take 8,000 IU of vitamin D3 daily for 4 weeks, then 4,000 IU daily for an additional 2 months. After the third month, recheck your blood level.
- If your vitamin D blood level is between 15.1 ng/ml (37.5 nmol/L) to 20 ng/ml (50 nmol/L) with a normal calcium level, I recommend you take 6,000 IU daily for 4 weeks, then 4,000 IU daily for 2 additional months. After the third month, recheck your blood levels.

- If your vitamin D level is between 20.1 ng/ml (50 nmol/L) to 32 ng/ml (80 nmol/L), I recommend you take 4,000 IU daily for 4 weeks, then 2,000 IU daily. Again, recheck your vitamin D blood levels after the 3rd month..

- What if your levels are above 32 ng/ml (80 nmol/L)? Great, you are almost there. I would try to get your vitamin D levels above 50 ng/ml (125 nmol/L) or even 60 to 100 ng/ml (150 to 250 nmol/L) for optimal health and disease prevention. I would recommend you take at least 2,000 IU daily of vitamin D3. Recheck your blood calcium and vitamin D levels after 3 months. If your vitamin D level is still below 50 ng/ml (125 nmol/L), consider increasing the dose to 4,000 IU daily or simply increase your time outdoors and lose the extra pounds.

It may take up to 1 year to optimize your vitamin D blood levels. Remember, life is a marathon and not a sprint. Be patient. The goal is to create a healthier, disease-resistant body that will allow you to enjoy the richness life has to offer. Supplementing a healthy diet with extra vitamin D is part of a holistic approach that will help you maintain healthier bones and prevent heart disease, diabetes, and, ultimately, cancer. Best of luck in your journey.

For information on where to buy vitamin D, visit your local community health food store and ask for vitamin D3. Also, see the listing in Appendix A of recommended online retailers of vitamin D3.

To get up to date information regarding vitamin D research, please visit our website www.vitaminD-prescription.com and join our email newsletter.

AUTHOR BIO

Dr. Eric Madrid completed his undergraduate work at the University of California Los Angeles (UCLA) where he earned his BS degree in Microbiology and Molecular Genetics. In 2002, he graduated from The Ohio State University School of Medicine where he earned his Doctorate of Medicine (MD) degree. He is Board Certified in Family Medicine and practices at Rancho Family Medical Group & Rancho Wellness Center, Temecula, Calif. Dr. Madrid and his wife, Whanda, have been married since 1998 and have 2 children. Dr. Madrid served 2 years as Chair Person for his local *Relay for Life,* sponsored by the American Cancer Society. He believes prevention is the best way to eliminate cancer and other diseases. Lifestyle and nutrition play a huge role in accomplishing this. Dr. Madrid also conducts product research and development for eHealthSupplies.com, an internet health portal.

GLOSSARY

Analogue- a type of molecule that is similar to the original. May also be a variation of the original molecule.

Bisphosphonates- A class of medicines used to treat osteoporosis. Examples include Boniva, Actonel and Fosamax.

Cholecalciferol- also known as vitamin D3. The form of vitamin D with maximal efficiency and potency.

Double Blind, Placebo controlled study- A study in which both the researchers and participants are unaware of who is getting the active drug/ supplement vs. the placebo

Enzyme- A protein which helps a biochemical reaction to occur.

Erogcalciferol- Also known as vitamin D2. Not as effective in treating clinical vitamin D deficiency but commonly found in multivitamins.

Hemoglobin A1C (HgA1C)- A blood test which provides an estimate of average blood sugar over the prior 3 months. Diabetic's goal is less than 7%. Non diabetics are between 4% and 6%.

Macrophages- A type of white blood cell which help "eat" bacteria and viruses that infect the blood.

MD- Doctor of Medicine degree, awarded to medical students upon completion of medical school.

PhD- Doctor of Philosophy. A degree given to scientists from various fields of study

Renin-a chemical which increases blood pressure.

ScD- Doctorate of Science degree.

T Cells- a type of white blood cell which helps the immune system.

BIBLIOGRAPHY

15 non dairy foods high in calcium. Accessed November 11, 2008 from http://www.healthdiaries.com/eatthis/15-non-dairy-foods-high-in-calcium.html.

58,800,000 million people die from heart disease worldwide. World Health Organization. Accessed November 11, 2008 from http://redwoodage.com/content/view/151525/45.

40% of people smoked in 1965 compared with 20.8% in 2003 according to Centers for Disease Control, Accessed January 12, 2008 from http://www.cdc.gov/nchs/data/hus/hus07.pdf#063

Adams, John S., and Gene Lee. 1997 (August). Gains in bone mineral density with resolution of vitamin D intoxication. *Annals of Internal Medicine* 127(3): 203-206.

Al Faraj, Saud, Khalaf Al Mutairi. 2003 (January). Vitamin D deficiency and chronic low back pain in Saudi Arabia. *Spine- An International Journal for the Study of the Spine* 28(2):177-179.

Al-Allaf, A.W., P.A. Mole, C.R. Paterson, and T. Pullar. 2003. Bone health in patients with fibromyalgia. *Rheumatology* 42: 1202-1206.

American Cancer Society website. Melanoma deadlier in blacks. Accessed October 26 2008 from http://www.cancer.org/docroot/NWS/content/NWS_1_1x_Melanoma_Deadlier_in_Blacks. asp.

American Diabetes Association. All about diabetes. Accessed September 30, 2008 from http://www.diabetes.org/about-diabetes.jsp.

Anu Prabhala, Rajesh Garg; and Paresh Dandona. Severe myopathy associated with vitamin D deficiency in western New York. *Archives of Internal Medicine* 160(8): .

Araugo, O. E., F. P. Flowers, K. Brown. 1991 (July-August). Vitamin D therapy and psoriasis. *DICP , The Annals of Pharmacoptherapy*, 25(7-8): 835-839.

Armas, Laura, B. Hollis, R. Heaney. Vitamin D2 is much less effective than vitamin d3 in humans. *Journal of Clinical Endocrinology & Metabolism* 89(11): 5387-5391.

Autier Philippe, Sara Gandini. 2007 (September). Vitamin D supplementation and total mortality: A meta-analysis of randomized controlled trials. *Archives of Internal Medicine* 167(16): 1730-1737

Belluck, Pam. 2005 (March). Children's life expectancy being cut short by obesity. *New York Times.* Accessed November 18, 2008 from http://www.nytimes.com/2005/03/17/health/17obese.htm.

Bertone-Johnson, Elizabeth, Wendy Y. Chen, Michael F. Holick, Bruce Hollis, et al. 2005 (August). Plasma 25-OH hydroxyvitamin D and 1,25- dihydroxyvitamin D and risk of breast cancer. *Cancer Epidemiology Biomarkers Prevention* 14(8): 1991-7.

Berube, Sylvie, Caroline Diorio, Benoit Massee, et al. 2005 (July). Vitamin D and calcium intakes from food or supplements and mammographic breast density. *Cancer Epidemiol Biomarkers Prev* 14(7): 1653-1659.

Berube, Sylvie, Caroline Diorio, Wendy Verhoek-Oftedahl, and Jacques Brisson, 2004. Vitamin D, calcium, and mammographic breast densities. *Cancer Epidemiol Biomarkers Prev* 13(9):1466-1472 .

Berwick, Marianne , Bruce K. Armstrong, Leah Ben-Porat, Judith Fine, Anne Kricker, Carey Eberle, and Raymond Barnhill. 2005. Sun exposure and mortality from melanoma. *Journal of the National Cancer Institute* 97(3):195-199.

Birge S. J., N. Morrow-Howell, E. K. Proctor. 1994. Hip fracture. *Clin Geriatrics Med* 10:589-609

Bischoff, Heike, B. Hannes, B. Stahelin, Walker Dick, et al. 2003 (November). Effects of vitamin D and calcium supplementation on falls: a randomized controlled trial. *Journal of Bone and Mineral Research* 18(2):343-351.

Bischoff-Ferrari, Heike, Walter C. Willett, DrPH; John B. Wong, MD; Edward, et. al. (2005) Fracture Prevention With Vitamin D Supplementation A Meta-analysis of Randomized Controlled Trials *JAMA.* 2005;293:2257-2264.

Bischoff-Ferrari, Heike, E. Giovannucci, W. Willetm, et al. 2006. Estimation of optimal serum concentrations of 25 hydroxyvitamin D for multiple health outcomes. *American Journal of Clinical Nutrition* 84: 18-24.

Blair, Debra. Byham-Gray, L, E. Lewis, S. McCaffrey. 2008. Prevalence of vitamin D deficiency and effects of supplementation with ergocalciferol (vitamin D2) in stage 5 chronic kidney disease patients. *Journal of Renal Nutrition* 18(4): 375-382.

Blackmore, K. M., M. Lesosky, and H. Barnett. 2008 (August). Vitamin D from dietary intake and sunlight exposure and the risk of hormone receptor defined breast cancer. *Am J Epidemiol* . 2008 Oct 15;168(8):915-24. Aug 27.

Blue Zones Community web site with Dr. Mehmet Oz. Accessed on November 25, 2008. from http://www.bluezones.com/

Bone mineral density in a racially and ethnically diverse group of men. *The Journal of Clinical Endocrinology & Metabolism* Vol. 93, No. 1 40-46.

Boniva, Highlights of prescribing information. Accessed on September 21, 2008 from http://www.rocheusa.com/products/Boniva/PI.pdf.

Boschert, Sherry. 2008. Vitamin D inadequacy might have a role in chronic pain. *Family Practice News* 38(3): 49.

Bostick, Roberd M, John D. Potter, T. A. Sellers. 2003, Relation of calcium, vitamin D, and dairy food intake to incidence of colon cancer among older women. *American Journal of Epidemiology* Vol. 137, No. 12: 1302-1317

Bray, George A., Samara Joy Nielsen, and Barry M. Popkin. 2004. Consumption of high fructose corn syrup in beverages may play a role in the obesity epidemic. *American Journal of Clinical Nutrition* 79: 537-543.

Brisson, Jacques, Sylvie Berube, Caroline Diorio, et al. 2007 (May). Synchronized seasonal variations of mammographic breast density and plasma 25-hydroxyvitamin D. *Cancer Epidemiology Biomarkers Prevention* 16(5): 929-933.

Buckley, Lenore M., Edward, D. Leib, Kathryn S. Catularo, Pamela M. Vacek, and Sheldon M. Cooper. 1996 (December). Calcium and vitamin D3 supplementation prevents bone loss in the spine secondary to low-dose corticosteroids in patients with rheumatoid arthritis: A randomized, double-blind, placebo controlled trial. *Annals of Internal Medicine* 125(12): 961-968.

Carter, Mary. 2006. Heart disease still the most likely reason you'll die. Accessed November 11, 2008 from http://www.cnn.com/2006/HEALTH/10/30/heart.overview/index.html.

Cancer Facts and FiguresCancer.org website: Cancer facts and figures. Accessed September 28, 2008 from http://www.cancer.org/downloads/STT/2008CAFFfinalsecured.pdf.

Cannell, J. J., B. W. Hollis, M. Zasloff, and R. P. Heaney. 2008 (January). Diagnosis and treatment of vitamin D deficiency. *Expert Opinion on Pharmacotherapy* 9: 107-118.

Cannell, J. J., R. Vieth, J. C. Umhau, M. F. Holick, W. B. Grant, S. Madronich, C. F. Garland, and E. Giovannucci. 2006. Epidemic influenza and vitamin D. *Epidemiology and Infection* 134: 1129-1140.

Cannell, J. J., Michael Zasloff, Cedric F. Garland, Robert Scragg, and Edward Giovannucci. 2008 (February). On the epidemiology of influenza. *Virology Journal* 5: 29. Available online http://www.virologyj.com/content/5/1/29

Centers for Disease Control and Prevention web site. Childhood obesity. *Healthy Youth*. Accessed October 29, 2008 from http://www.cdc.gov/HealthyYouth/obesity/index.htm.

Cervical cancer is the 2nd leading cancer worldwide. Accessed November 26, 2008 from http://www.cervicalcancer.org/statistics.html.

Cervical cancer kills about 270,000 women each year. Accessed November 28, 2008 from http://www.cancer.gov/clinicaltrials/results/HPV-vaccine0406.

Chantal, Mathieu, Klaus Badenhoop.2005 (August). Vitamin D and type 1 diabetes mellitus; state of the art. *Trends in Endocrinology and Metabolism* 16(6): .

Chantal, Mathieu, C. Gysemans, A. Giulietti, and R.Bouillon. 2005. Vitamin D and diabetes. *Diabetologia* 48: 1247-1257.

Chen, Wendy Y., Elizabeth R. Bertone-Johnson, David J. Hunter, Walter C. Willet, and Susan E. Hankinson. 2005 (October). Associations between polymorphisms in the vitamin D receptor and breast cancer risk. *Cancer Epidemiology Biomarkers Prevention* 14(10): .

Chiu, Graham. 2005 (November). Vitamin D deficiency among patients attending a central New Zealand rheumatology outpatient clinic. *Journal of the New Zealand Medical Association* 118(1225)

Cho, Eunyoung, Donna Spiegelman, David J. Hunter, et al. 2003 (August). Premenopausal intakes of vitamin a, c and e, folate and carotenoids, and risk of breast cancer. *Cancer Epidemiology, Biomarkers & Prevention* 12: 713.

Cigolini, Massimo, Maria Pina Iagulli, Valentino Miconi, Micaela Galiotto, Simonetta Lombardi, Giovanni Targher. 2006 (March). Serum 25-hydroxyvitamin D3 concentrations and prevalence of cardiovascular disease among type 2 diabetic patients. Diabetes Care 29(3): .

Clark, L. C., G. F. Combs, B. W. Turnbull, E. H. Slate, D. K. Chalker. 1996. Effects of selenium supplementation for cancer prevention in patients with carcinoma of the skin. A randomized controlled trial. Nutritional Prevention of Cancer Study Group. *JAMA*.

Colston, K W, M. J. Colston, and D. Feldman. 1,25-dihydroxyvitamin D3 and malignant melanoma: the presence of receptors and inhibition of cell growth in culture. *Endocrinology* 108: 1083-1086.

Cox M. D., and John G. Haddard Malcolm. 1984 (November). Lymphoma, hypercalcemia and the sunshine vitamin. *Annals of Internal Medicine* 121(9): 709-712.

Dale Kiefer. 2007 (February). Unraveling a centuries-old mystery why is flu risk so much higher in the winter? *Life Extension Magazine*. Accessed on Dec. 11. 2009 from www.lef.org/magazine/mag2007/feb2007_report_vitamind_01.htm.

Datta, S., M. Alfaham, D.P. Davies, F. Dunstan, S. Woodhead, J. Evans, and B. Richards. 2002. Vitamin D deficiency in pregnant women from a non-European ethnic minority population, an interventional study BJOG. *International Journal of Obstetrics & Gynaecology* 109(8): 905-908.

Dawson-Hughes, Bess. Susan S. Harris., Elizabeth A. Krall, and Gerard R. Dallal. 1997 (September). Effect of calcium and vitamin D supplementation on bone density in men and women 65 years of age or older. *New England Journal of Medicine* 337(10): 670-676.

de Boer, Ian H., Lesley F. Tinker, Stephanie Connelly, J. David Curb, Barbara V. Howard. 2008 (January). Calcium plus vitamin D supplementation and the risk of incident diabetes in the women's health initiative. *Diabetes Care* 31: 701-707.

Dennis, Leslie K.; Laura E. Beane Freeman; and Marta J. VanBeek. 2003 (December). Sunscreen use and the risk for melanoma: a quantitative review. *Annals of Internal Medicine* 139(12): 966-978.

Diagnosed with breast cancer at 21: A survivor's story. Accessed October 4th, 2008 from http://www.foxnews.com/story/0,2933,351378,00.html.

Di Cesar, David J., Robert Ploutz-Snyder, Ruth S. Weinstock, and Arnold M. Moses. Vitamin D deficiency is more common in type 2 than in type 1 diabetes. (2006) *Diabetes Care* 29: 174

Dietary Reference Intakes (DRIs): Recommended Intakes for Individuals, Vitamins Food and Nutrition Board, Institute of Medicine, National Academy. Accessed April 12, 2008 from http://www.iom.edu/Object.File/Master/21/372/0.pdf.

Digestive System Image taken from NIH, National Digestive Diseases Information Clearing House. Accessed January 12, 2009 http://digestive.niddk.nih.gov/ddiseases/pubs/yrdd/images/digest.gif

Double Helix- 50 years of DNA. *Nature Online.* Accessed November 14' 2008 from http://www.nature.com/nature/dna50/.

Egsmose, Charlotte, Birger Lund, Peter McNair, et al. 1987. Low serum levels of 25-hydroxyvitamin D and 1,25- di-hydroxyvitamin D in institutionalized old people: Influence of solar exposure and Vitamin D supplementation. *Age and Ageing* 16: 35-40.

FDA States Gardasil associated with 20 deaths. Accessed September 22, 2008 from http://www.fda.gov/CBER/safety/gardasil071408.htm.

Feskanich, Diane, Jing Ma, C. S. Fuchs, et al. 2004 (September). Plasma vitamin D metabolites and risk of colorectal cancer in women. *Cancer Epidemiology Biomarkers Prevention* 13: 9. September 2004

Feskanich, Diane, Walter C. Willet, and Graham A. Colditz. 2003. Calcium, vitamin D, milk consumption, and hip fractures: a prospective study among postmenopausal women. *American Journal Of Clinical Nutrition* 77:504-511.

Finley, John W., Ip Clement, Donald J. Lisk, et al. 2001. Cancer-protective properties of high-selenium broccoli. *J. Agric. Food Chem* 49(5): 2679-2683.

Fleming discovers Penicillin. Accessed October 13th 2008 from http://history1900s.about.com/od/medicaladvancesissues/a/penicillin_2.htm.

Flicker, Leon, Robert J. MacInnis, G. Dip Biostat, et al. 2005. Should older people in residential care receive vitamin D to prevent falls? Results of randomized trial. *Journal of the American Geriatrics Society* 53:1881-1888.

Flicker L, Mead K, MacInnis RJ, Nowson C, et al. 2003 Serum vitamin D and falls in older women in residential care in Australia. *J Am Geriatr Soc,* 51(11):1533-8.

Forman, John P., Heike A. Bischoff-Ferrari, Walter C. Millet, Meir J. Stampfer, and Gary C. Curhan. 2005. Vitamin D intake and risk of incident hypertension: Results from three large prospective cohort studies. *Hypertension Journal of the American Heart Association* 46: 676-682.

Forman, John P., Edward Giovannucci, Michelle D. Holmes, Heike A. Bischoff-Ferrari, et al. 2007. Plasma 25-hydroxyvitamin D levels and risk of incident hypertension. *Hypertension Journal of the American Heart Association* 49; 1063-1069.

Forouhi, Nita G., Jian'an Luan, Andrew Cooper, Barbara J. Boucher, and Nicholas J. Wareham. 2008 Baseline serum 25-hydroxyvitamin D is predictive of future glycemic status and insulin resistance. *Diabetes* 57:2619-2625.

Fosamax drug sales: Source (http://www.wikinvest.com/concept/Osteo-porosis_drug_market. Permission for use granted by Conrad Parker of wikinvest.com.

Freedman, D. M., M. Dosemeci, and K. McGlyn. 2002. Sunlight and mortality from breast, ovarian, colon, prostate and non-melanoma skin cancer: a composite death certificate based case-control study, *Occupational and Environmental Medicine* 59:259-262.

Friedrich M., C. Villena-Heinsen, R. Axt-Fliedner, R. Meyberg, W. Tilgen, W. Schmidt, and J. Reichrath. 2002 (January-February). Analysis of 25-hydroxyvitamin D3-1alpha-hydroxylase in cervical tissue. *Anticancer Res* 22(1A):183-6.

Garland, Cedric, F. and Frank C. Garland. 1980 Do sunlight and vitamin d reduce the likelihood of colon cancer? *International Journal of Epidemiology* 9(3): 227-231.

Garland C., F. Garland, E. Gorham. 1992 (April). Could sunscreens increase melanoma risk? *Am J Public Health* 82(4): 614–5.

Garland C. F., Edward D. Gohram, Sharif B. Mohr, et al. 2007 (March). Vitamin D and prevention of breast cancer: Pooled analysis. *Journal of Steroid Biochemistry and Molecular Biology* 103(3-5): 708-711.

Garland, C, R. B. Shekelle, E. Barrett-Connor, et al. 1985 (February). Dietary vitamin D and calcium and risk of colorectal cancer: A 19 year prospective study in men. *The Lancet* 1(8424):307-9.

Genetic Mutations explains the difference between skin pigmentation. Accessed October 19, 2008 from http://www.washingtonpost.com/wpdyn/content/article/2005/12/15/AR2005121501728pf.html.

Giovannucci, Edward, Yan Lui, Bruce Hollis, Eric B. Rimm. 2008 (June). 25-hydroxvitamin D and risk of myocardial infarction in men. *Archives of Internal Medicine* 168(11): .

Giovannucci, Edward, Y. Lui, E. Rimm, et al. 2006 (April). Prospective study of predictors of vitamin D status and cancer incidence and mortality in men. *Journal of the National Institute* 98(7): 451-459.

Giovannucci, Edward, Yan Liu, and Walter C. Willet. 2006 (December Cancer incidence and mortality and vitamin D in black and white male health professionals. *Cancer Epidemiology Biomarkers Prevention* 2006; 15(15):12.

Gisondi, Paolo, Micol Del Giglio, Vincenzo Di Francesco, Mauro Zamboni, and Giampiero Girolomioni. 2008: Weight loss improves the response of obese patients with moderate to severe chronic plaque psoriasis to low dose cyclosporine therapy: A randomized, controlled, investigator-blinded clinical trial. *American Journal Clinical Nutrition* 88: 1242-1247.

Glerup H., K. Mikkelsen, L. Poulsen, E. Hass, S. Overbeck, J. Thomsen, P. Charles, E. F. Eriksen. 2000. Commonly recommended daily intake of vitamin D is not sufficient if sunlight exposure is limited. *J Intern Med* 2000 247: 260–268.

Global cancer rates could increase by 50% to 15 million. World Health Organization website. Accessed November 26, 2008 from http://www.who.int/mediacentre/news/releases/2003/pr27/en/.

Gordon Catherine M., Kerrin C. DePeter, Henry A. Feldman, Grace Estherann, and S. Jean Emans. 2004. Prevalence of Vitamin D deficiency among healthy adolescents. *Arch Pediatr Adolesc Med* 158:531-537.

Gordon, Serena. 2008 (June 3). Vitamin D Deficiency Deficiency Puts puts 40% of U.S. Infants and Toddlers At at Risk. *Washington Post*. Accessed on September 24, 2008 from http://www.washingtonpost.com/wp-dyn/content/article/2008/06/03/AR2008060301125.html.

Gorham, Edward, Frank C. Garland, and Cedric F. Garland. 1990 Sunlight and breast cancer incidence in the USSR. *International Journal of Epidemiology* 19(4): 820-824

Goswami, R., S. K. Mishra, and N. Kochupillai. 2008. Prevalence & potential significance of vitamin D deficiency in Asian Indians. *Indian J Med Res* March: 229-238.

Gorham, Edward D., C. F. Garland, F. C. Garland, et al. 2005 (October). Vitamin D and prevention of colorectal cancer. *Journal of Steroid Biochemistry and Molecular Biology* 97(1-2): 179-194.

Gorham, Edward D., Cedric Garland, F. Garland, et al. 2007. Optimal vitamin D status for colorectal cancer prevention: A quantitative meta analysis. *American Journal of Preventive Medicine* 32(3): .

Grace, S., Jean Emans. 2004. Prevalence of vitamin D deficiency among healthy adolescents. *Arch Pediatr Adolesc Med* 158: 531-537.

Grant, William B. 2002 (March). An Estimate of premature cancer mortality in the U.S. due to inadequate doses of solar ultraviolet-b radiation. *Cancer* 94(6): 1867-1875.

Gray, Denis Pereira. (2003) (November) Robert Edgar Hope-Simpson. *British Medical Journal*. Accessed January 4, 2009 from http://www.pubmedcentral.nih.gov/articlerender.fcgi?artid=261759.

Greer, Frank, 2008. AAP -New guidelines double the amount of recommended vitamin D. *American Academy of Pediatrics* web site -October 13, 2008. Accessed on October 24, 2008 from http://www.aap.org/pressroom/nce/nce08vitamind.htm.

HannannMarian T.,HeatherJ.Litman,AndreB.Araujo,ChristineE.McLennan, Robert R. McLean, John B. McKinlay, Tai C. Chen, and Michael F. Holick Serum 25-Hydroxyvitamin hydroxyvitamin D and bone mineral density in a racially and ethnically diverse group of men. *The Journal of Clinical Endocrinology & Metabolism* 93(1): 40-46.

Haole Li, Meir J. Stampfer, J. Bruce Hollis, et al. 2007 (March). A prospective study of plasma vitamin d metabolites, vitamin D receptor polymorphisms, and prostate cancer. *PLOS Medicine* 4(3): 0562-0571.

Harper, Diane. As quoted on the website Alliance of Human Research Protection. Accessed January 12, 2009. http://www.ahrp.org/cms/content/view/503/27/

Harris, Susan S. Symposium: 2006 (April). Optimizing Vitamin vitamin D intake for populations with special needs: Barriers to effective food fortification and supplementation vitamin D and African Americans. *Journal. Nutrition.* 136:1126-1129.

Harris Susan S., Bess Dawson-Hughes, and Gayle A. Perrone. 1999. Plasma25-hydroxyvitamin D responses of younger and older men to three weeks of supplementation with 1800 IU/day of vitamin D. *Journal of the American College of Nutrition* 18(5):470-474.

Harris, Susan S., Elpidoforos Soteriades, Jo Anna Stina Coolidge, Sharmilla Mudgal, and Bess Dawson-Hughes. Vitamin D insufficiency and hyperparathyroidism in a low income, multiracial, elderly population. *Journal of Clinical Endocrinology & Metabolism* 85(11): 4125-4130.

Hartge, Patricia, Unhee Lim, D. Michael Freedman, et al. 2006. Ultraviolet radiation, dietary vitamin D, and risk of non-Hodgkin lymphoma (United States). *Cancer Causes Control* 17: 1045-1052.

Hathcock, John N., Andrew Shao, Reinhold Vieth, and Robert Heaney. 2007. Risk assessment for vitamin D. *American Journal of Clinical Nutrition* 85: 6-18.

Hayes, Colleen E. (2000). Vitamin D: a natural inhibitor of multiple sclerosis. *Proceedings of the Nutrition Society* 59: 531-535.

Hayes, Colleen E., M. T. Cantorna, and H. F. DeLuca. 1997. Vitamin D and multiple sclerosis. *Proceedings of the Society for Experimental Biology and Medicine* 216: 21-27.

HealthandSurvival.com website. Haiti: Mud cakes become staple diet as cost of food soars beyond a family's reach. Accessed November 14, 2008 from http://healthandsurvival.com/2008/07/29/haiti-mud-cakes-become-staple-diet-as-cost-of-food-soars-beyond-a-familys-reach.

Heike A. Bischoff-Ferrari, Walter C. Willett, John B. Wong, Edward Giovannucci, Thomas Dietrich, Bess Dawson-Hughes. 2005 (May). Fracture prevention with vitamin D supplementation: A meta-analysis of Randomized controlled trials. *JAMA* 293(18):2257-2264 .

Holick, Michael F., 2002 (July). Too little vitamin D in pre-menopausal women: Why Should We Care? *American Journal of Clinical Nutrition,* Vol 76, No.(1,): 3-4, July 2002.

Holick, Michael F. 2005. The vitamin D epidemic and its health consequences. *American Society for Nutrition* 2739S-2748S.

Holland, D. B., E. J. Wood, S. G. Roberts, M. R. West, W. J. Cunliffe. 1989. Epidermal keratin levels during oral 1-alpha-hydroxyvitamin D3 treatment for psoriasis. *Skin Pharmacology* 2(2):68-76.

Hsia, Judith, Gerardo Heiss, Hong Ren, Matthew Allison, et al. 2007. Calcium/vitamin D supplementation and cardiovascular events. *Circulation* 115: 846-854.

Huisman, A. M., K. P. White, A. Algra, M. Harth, R. Vieth, J. W. Jacobs, J. W. Bijlsma, D. A. Bell. 2001 (November). Vitamin D levels in women with systemic lupus erythematosus and fibromyalgia. *J Rheumatol* 28(11): 2535-9.

Hutchinson, Peter, Joy E. Osborne, John T. Lear, Andrew G. Smith, P. William Bowers, Paul N. Morris, Peter W. Jones, Christopher York, Richard C. Strange, and Anthony A. Fryer. 2000 (February). Vitamin D receptor polymorphisms are associated with altered prognosis in patients with malignant melanoma. *Clinical Cancer Research* 6: 498–504.

Hyppönem, Elina, Esa Laara, Antii Reunanen, Marjo-Riitta Jarvelin, and Suvi M. Virtanen. 2001. Intake of vitamin D and risk of type 1 diabetes: a birth-cohort. *Lancet* 358: 1500-1503.

Hyponnen, Elina, and Chris Power. 2006 (October). Vitamin D status and glucose homeostasis in the 1958 British birth cohort. *Diabetes Care* 29(10):2244-2246 .

IncredibleEdd.org website. Nutrient content of a large egg. Accessed November 28, 2008 from http://www.incredibleegg.org/pdf/Nutrient_Content_Large_Egg.pdf.

Ingles, Sue Ann. 2008 Can diet and/or sunlight modify the relationship between vitamin D receptor polymorphisms and prostate cancer risk? *Nutrition Reviews* 65(8): S105-S107.

Ingles, Sue Ann, Ronal K. Ross, Mimi C. Yu, et al. 1997 (January). Association of prostate cancer risk with genetic polymorphisms in vitamin D receptor and androgen receptor. *Journal of the National Cancer Institute* 89(2): 166-170.

Jackson, C., S. Gaugris, S.S. Sen, and D. Hosking, 2007. The effect of cholecalciferol (vitamin D3) on the risk of fall and fracture. QJM 100(4):185-192

Jackson, Rebecca D.. Andrea Z. LaCroix, Margery Gass, Robert B. Wallace, John Robbins, et al. 2006 (February). Calcium plus Vitamin D supplementation and the risk of fractures. New England Journal of Medicine. 354: 7.

Jacobs, Elizabeth T., and David Alberts, David. 2008. Vitamin D insufficiency in southern Arizona- Americans. *Journal of Clinical Nutrition* 2008; 87: 608-613.

Javaid, M. K., S. R. Crozier, N. C. Harvey. 2006 (January). Maternal vitamin D status during pregnancy and childhood bone mass at age 9 years: a longitudinal study. *The Lancet* 367(9504): 36-43.

John, Ester M., Gary G. Schwartz, Darlene M. Dreon, and Jocelyn Koo. 1999 (May). Vitamin D and breast cancer risk: The NHANES I epidemiologic follow up study, 1971-1975 to 1992. *Cancer Epidemiology, Biomarkers & Prevention* 8: 399-406.

John, Esther, Gary Schwartz, Jocelyn Koo, and David Can Den Berg. 2005 (June). Sun exposure, vitamin d receptor gene polymorphisms, and risk of advanced prostate cancer. *Cancer Research* 65(12): 5470-5479.

Judd, Suzanne E., Mark S. Nanes, Thomas R. Ziegler, Peter WF Wilson, and Vin Tangpricha. 2008. Optimal vitamin D status attenuates the age-associated increase in systolic blood pressure in white Americans: Results from the third National Health and Nutrition Examination Survey. *American Journal of Clinical Nutrition* 87:136-141.

Kamen, Diane, G. Cooper, H. Bouali, et al. 2006 (February). Vitamin D deficiency in systemic lupus erythematosus. *Autoimmunity Review* 5(2): 114-117. Lemire, Jacques M., Ann Ince, Masayoshi Takashima. 1992. 1,25-dihydroxyvitamin D3 attenuates of expression of experimental murine lupus of MRL/1 mice. *Autoimmunity* 12(2): 143-48.

Klontz, Karl C., and David W. Acheson. 2007 (July). *Food and Drug Administration.* Dietary supplement vitamin D intoxication correspondence. *New England Journal of Medicine* 357: 308-309.

Knight, Julia A., Maia Lesosky, Heidi Barnett, Janet M. Raboud, and Reinhold Vieth. 2007 (March). Vitamin D and reduced risk of breast cancer: A population-based case-control study. *Cancer Epidemiology, Biomarkers & Prevention* 16(3): 422-429.

Krishnan, Aruna, Jacqueline Moreno, Larisa Nonn, et al. 2007. Novel pathways that contribute to the anti-proliferative and chemopreventive activities of calcitrol in prostate cancer. *Journal of Steroid Biochemistry & Molecular Biology* 103: 694-702.

Kumaravel Rajakumar. 2003. Vitamin D, cod-liver oil, sunlight, and rickets: A historical perspective. *Pediatrics* 112: e132-e135. Mejia, Luis. Fortification of foods: Historical development and current practices.

Accessed September 22, 2008 from (http://www.unu.edu/unupress/food/8F154e/8F154E03.htm

Kumaravel Rajakumar, and Stephen B. Thomas. 2005. Reemerging nutritional rickets: A historical perspective. *Arch Pediatr Adolesc Med* *159(4):* 335-341.

Lajous, Martin, Eduardo Lazcano-Ponce, Mauricio Hernandez-Avila, Walter Willett, and Isabelle Romieu. 2006 (March). Folate, vitamin B6 and B12 intake and the risk of breast cancer among Mexican women. *Cancer Epidemiology& Biomarkers Prevention* 15(3): 443-448.

Lane, Nancy E. L. Robert Gore , Steven R. Cummings, Marc C. Hochberg, Jean C. Scott , Elizabeth N. Williams, and Michael C. Nevitt. 2001 (March). Study of osteoporotic fractures research group serum vitamin D levels and incident changes of radiographic hip osteoarthritis: A longitudinal study. *Arthritis & Rheumatism* 42(5): 854 – 860.

Lappe, Joan M., Dianne Travers-Gustafson, K. Michael Davies, Robert R. Recker, and Robert P. Heany. 2007. Vitamin D and calcium supplementation reduces cancer risk: results of a randomized trial. *American Journal of Clinical Nutrition* 85:6 1586-1591.

LeBlanc, Adrian, Victor Schneider, Jean Krebs, Harlan Evan, Satish Jhingran, and Phillip Johnson 1987 November). Spinal bone mineral after 5 weeks of bed rest. *Calcified Tissue International* 41(5):

LeBlanc, Adrian, Victor Schneider, Jean Krebs, Harlan Evan, Satish Jhingran, and Phillip Johnson 1987 Lee, Joyce M., Jessica R. Smith, Barbara L. Phillip, et al. 2007 (January). Vitamin D deficiency in a healthy group of mothers and newborn infants. *Clinical Pediatrics* 46(1): 42-44.

Lefkowitz, Ellen Schneider, and Cedric F. Garland. Sunlight, vitamin D and ovarian cancer mortality rates in US women. *International Journal of Epidemiology* 23(6): 1133-1136.

Lips, Paul. Vitamin D deficiency and secondary hyperparathyroidism in the elderly: Consequences for bone loss and fractures and therapeutic implications. *Endocrine Reviews* 22(4): 477-501.

Lips, Paul, Wilco C. Graafmans, Marcel E. Ooms, P. Dick Bezemer, Lex Bouter. 1996 (February). Vitamin D supplementation and fracture incidence in elderly persons 124(4): 400-406.

Li. Yan Chun. 2003. Vitamin D regulation of the renin-angiotensin system. *Journal of Cellular Biochemistry* 88: 327-331.

Li, Yan Chun, Juan Kong, Minjie Wei, Zhou-Feng Chen, Shu Q. Liu, and Li-Ping Cao. 2002 (July). 1,25- dihydroxyvitamin D3 is a negative endocrine regulator of the renin-angiotensin system. *Journal of Clinical Investigation* 110(2): 229-238

Lyman, David. 2005 (January). Undiagnosed Vitamin D Deficiency in the Hospitalized Patient. *American Family Physician* 299-304.

MacNeil, Jane Salodof. 2008 (June). Low vitamin D levels may explain pediatric pain. *Family Practice News 38(11): 24.*

Mahoney, Diana. 2008 (February). Disability seems worse in RA Patients with low vitamin D. *Family Practice News,* page 33 Accessed on December 11, 2008 from http://download.journals.elsevierhealth.com/pdfs/journals/0300-7073/PIIS0300707308702391.pdf

Marcus, Mary Brophy. 2008 (June 6). Lack of Vitamin D rampant in infant and teens. *USA Today.*. Accessed September, 24, 2008 from http://www. usatoday.com/news/health/2008-06-16-vitamin-d-main_N.htm.

Martinez, Elena, W. C. Willet. 1998 (February). Calcium, vitamin D, and colorectal cancer: a review of the epidemiologic evidence. *Cancer Epidemiology, Biomarkers & Prevention* 7: 163–168.

Mathieu, Chantal, and Klaus Badenhoop. 2005 (August). Vitamin D and type 1 diabetes mellitus; state of the art. *Trends in Endocrinology and Metabolism* 16(6):261–266

McAlindon, Timothy E., David T. Felson, Yuqing Zhang, et al. 1996 (September). Relation of dietary intake and serum levels of vitamin D to progression of osteoarthritis of the knee among participants in the Framingham study. *Annals of Internal Medicine* 125(5): 353–359.

McGartland, C., P. J. Robson, L. Murray, G. Cran, M. J. Savage, D. Watkins, M. Rooney, and C. Boreham. **2003** (September). Carbonated soft drink consumption and bone mineral density in adolescence: The Northern Ireland Young Hearts project. *Journal of Bone and Mineral Research*, 18:1563-1569 doi: 10.1359/jbmr.2003.18.

McJunkin, Melissa. 2007 (October). andMSG: The hidden cause for weight gain. Accessed November 29, 2008 from http://www.associatedcontent.com/article/431809/msg_the_hidden_cause_for_weight_gain. html?cat=5 (accessed November 29th 2008)

Melamed, M. H. S., Michael L. Eric, D. Michos, Wendy Post, Brad Astor. 2008. 25-hydroxyvitamin D levels and the risk of mortality in the general population. *Archives of Internal Medicine* 168(15): 1629-1637.

Melamed, Michal L., Paul Muntner, Erin D. Michos, et al. 2008. Serum 25-hydroxyvitamin D levels and the prevalence of peripheral arterial disease. *Arteriosclerosis, Thrombosis and Vascular Biology* 28: 1179.

Melanoma far more deadly in African Americans. Accessed October 26, 2008 from http://www.cancer.org/docroot/NWS/content/NWS_1_1x_Melanoma_Deadlier_in_Blacks.asp

Melanoma incidence. National Cancer Institute. Accessed October 19, 2008 from http://www.cancer.gov/cancertopics/types/melanoma.

Melanoma incidence worldwide. Accessed October 19, 2008 from http://en.wikipedia.org/wiki/Melanoma.

Melanoma, What Causes It? According to the *American Cancer Society*. Revised 7/01/08. Accessed website January 20, 2009. http://www.cancer.org/docroot/CRI/content/CRI_2_2_2X_What_causes_melanoma_skin_cancer_50.asp

Merck Manual, Vitamin Deficiency, Dependency and Toxicity. Pages 41–44. 18th edition, 2006.

Merewood, Anne, D. Supriya, C. Tai, Howard Bauchner, and Michael F. Holick. 2008. Association between vitamin d deficiency and primary cesarean section *Journal of Clinical Endocrinology & Metabolism* 10(1210): 2008-1217.

Michael F. 2002 (February). Vitamin D: the underappreciated D-lightful hormone that is important for skeletal and cellular health: **Multihormonal systems disorders**. *Current Opinion in Endocrinology & Diabetes* 9(1):87-98.

Michos, Erin D, Michal L. Melamed, Wendy Post, and Brad C. Astor. 2007. 25-OH vitamin D deficiency and the risk of all-cause mortality in the general population: Results from the third national health and nutrition examination survey linked mortality data. *Circulation,* 116: 826.

Mizoue, Tetsuya. 2004 (November). Ecological study of solar radiation and cancer mortality in Japan. *Health Physics* 87(5): 532-538.

Moan, Johan, Alina Carmen Porohnicu, Arne Dahlback, and Richard Setlow. 2008 (January). Addressing the health benefits and risks, involving vitamin D or skin cancer, of increased sun exposure. *PNAS* 105(2): 668-673.

Morimoto, S., K. Yoshikawa, T. Kozuka, Y. Kitano, S. Imanaka, K. Fukuo, E. Koh, and Y. Kumahara. 1986. An open study of vitamin D3 treatment in psoriasis vulgaris. *British Journal of Dermatology* 115: 421-429.

Morimoto, S., and Y. Kumahara. 1985. A patient with psoriasis cured by 1α-hydroxyvitamin D3. *Medical Journal of Osaka University* 35: 51-54.

Morimoto S, and Y. Yoshikawa. 1989 K. Psoriasis and vitamin D3: A review of our experience. *Arch Dermatol;* 125:231-234

Mother's vitamin d status during pregnancy will affect her baby's dental health. 2008. *Science Daily.* Accessed January 10, 2009 from http://www.sciencedaily.com/releases/2008/07/080704104315.htm.

MSG and use linked to obesity. *ScienceDaily.* Accessed November 29, 2008 from its influence on obesity: http://www.sciencedaily.com/releases/2008/08/080813164638.htm.

Muhe, Lulu, Sileshi Lulseged, Karen E. Mason, and Eric A. F. Simoes. 1997 (June). Case-control study of the role of nutritional rickets in the risk of developing pneumonia in Ethiopian children. *The Lancet* 349(9068): 1801–1804.

Multiple Sclerosis definition. Accessed November 25, 2008 from http://www.nationalmssociety.org.

Munger, Kassandra L.; Lynn I. Levin; Bruce W. Hollis; Noel S. Howard; Alberto Ascherio. 2006. Serum 25-hydroxyvitamin D levels and risk of multiple sclerosis *JAMA* 296: 2832-2838.

Munger, K.L., S. M. Zhang, E. O'Reilly, M. A. Hernán, M. J. Olek, W. C. Willett, and A. Ascherio. 2004. Vitamin D intake and incidence of multiple sclerosis. *American Academy of Neurology* 62: 60-65.

National Human Genome Research Institute web site: 2007 (October). A guide to your genome? *NIH Publication*. Accessed November 28' 2008 from http://www.genome.gov/Pages/Education/AllAboutthe HumanGenomeProject/GuidetoYourGenome07.pdf.

National Osteoporosis Foundation web site. Risk factors for osteoporosis. Accessed October 27, 2008 from http://www.nof.org/osteoporosis/diseasefacts.htm.

National Osteoporosis Foundation web site. Osteoporosis: Bone density. Accessed January 3, 2009 from http://www.nof.org/osteoporosis/bonemass.htm.

National PBM Drug Monograph Quadrivalent Human Papillomavirus (Types 6, 11, 16 18) Recombinant Vaccine (Gardasil®). VHA Pharmacy Benefits Management Strategic Healthcare Group and the Medical Advisory Panel February 2007. Accessed 01/20/2009 at http://www.pbm.va.gov/monograph/Gardasil.pdf

Nation Institutes of Health web site: Dietary Supplement Fact Sheet: Vitamin D. Accessed September 30, 2008 from http://ods.od.nih.gov/factsheets/vitamind.asp

Ng K, J. A. Meyerhardt, and K. Wu. 2008. Circulating 25-hydroxyvitamin D levels and survival in patients with colorectal cancer. *Journal of Clinical Oncology* 26: 2984–91.

Nicola Di Daniele, Maria Grazia Carbonelli, Nicola Candeloro, et. al (2004) Effect of supplementation of calcium and Vitamin D on bone mineral density and bone mineral content in peri- and post-menopause women: A double-blind, randomized, controlled trial. *Pharmacological Research* 50(6):637-641.

Nieves, J., F. Cosman, J. Herbert, V. Shen, and R. Lindsay. 1994. High prevalence of vitamin D deficiency and reduced bone mass in multiple sclerosis. *Neurology* 44:1687.

Nonn, Larisa, Lihong Peng, David Feldman, and Donna M. Peehl. 2006 (April). Inhibition of p38 by Vitamin D reduces interleukin-6 production in normal prostate cancer cells via mitogen activiated protein kinase phosphatase 5: Implication for prostate cancer prevention by vitamin D. *Cancer Res* 66(8): A516-4524.

Norman, Anthony, 2008. From vitamin D to hormone D: fundamentals of the vitamin D endocrine system essential for good health. *American Journal Clinical Nutrition* 88: 491S-499.

Ntais, Christos, Anastasia Polycarpou, and John P. A. Ioannidis. 2003 (December). Vitamin D receptor gene polymorphisms and risk of prostate cancer: A meta analysis. *Cancer Epidemiology, Biomarkers & Prevention* 12: 1395–1402.

Nursyam E. W., A. Amin, and C. M. Rumende. 2006 (January – March). The effect of vitamin D as supplementary treatment in patients with moderately advanced pulmonary tuberculous lesions. *Acta Med Indonesia* 38(1): 3-5.

Osteopenia definition: Accessed October 17, 2008: from http://www.medterms.com/script/main/art.asp?articlekey=8048.

Osteoporosis definition: Accessed October 17, 2008 from http://www.nof.org/osteoporosis/index.htm.

Osteoporosis drug market. Accessed October 18, 2008 from (http://www.wikinvest.com/concept/Osteoporosis_drug_market.

Palmer, Suetonia C., David O. McGregor, Petra Macaskill. 2007. Meta-analysis: Vitamin D compounds in chronic kidney disease. *Annals of Internal Medicine* 147: 840-853

Pfeifer, Michael, Bettina Begerow, Helmutt W. Minne, et al. 2000 (November). Effects of a short term vitamin D and calcium supplementation on body sway and secondary hyperparathyroidism in elderly women. *Journal of Bone and Mineral Research* 15:

Pilz, Stefan, Harald Dobnig, Brigitte Winklhofer-Roob, et al. 2008 (May). Low serum levels of 25-hydroxyvitamin D predict fatal cancer in patients referred to coronary angiography. *Cancer Epidemiology Biomarkers & Prevention* 17(5): 1228-33.

Pilz, Stefan, Winifred Marz, Britta Wellnitz, et al. (2008) Association of Vitamin D deficiency with heart failure and sudden cardiac death in a large cross sectional study of patients referred to coronary angiography. *Journal of Clinical Endocrinology & Metabolism* 93(10): 3927-3935

Plotnikoff , G. A., and J. M. Quigley. 2003 (December). Prevalence of severe hypovitaminosis D in patients with persistent, nonspecific musculoskeletal pain. *Mayo Clin Proc* 78(12):1463-70.

Pittas, Anastassios G., Bess Dawson-Hughes, Tricia Li, Rob M. Van Dam, Walter C. Willett, Joann E. Manson, and Frank B. Hu. 2006. Vitamin D and calcium intake in relation to type 2 diabetes in women. *Diabetes Care* 29(3): 650-656.

Porojnicu, Alina Carmen, Zoya Lagunova, Trude Eid Robsahm, et al. 2007 (May). Changes in risk of death from breast cancer with season and latitude. *Breast Cancer Research and Treatment* 102(3): 323-328.

Porthouse, Jill, Sarah Cockayne, Christine King, Lucy Saxon, et al. 2005. Randomised controlled trial of calcium and supplementation with cholecalciferol (vitamin D3) for prevention of fractures in primary care. *British Medical Journal* 330: 1030.

Powell, Alvin. Vitamin D critical to human TB response- *Findings illuminate possible prevention pathways (2006). Accessed Feb 1, 2009* ml http://www.news.harvard.edu/gazette/2006/03.09/01-tb.html

Probability of Developing Cancer. DevCan: Probability of Developing or Dying of Cancer Software, Version 6.2.1 Statistical Research and Applications Branch, National Cancer Institute, 2007. http://srab.cancer.gov/devcan. http://www.cancer.org/docroot/MIT/content/MIT_3_2X_Costs_of_Cancer.asp)

Purdue, Mark P., Patricia Hartge, Scott Davis, et al. 2007. Sun exposure, vitamin D receptor gene polymorphisms and risk of non-Hodgkin lymphoma. *Cancer Causes Control* 18: 989-999.

Roni Caryn Rabin, Vitamin D Deficiency May Lurk in Babies, 2008, New York Times, accessed August 29th, 2008, http://www.nytimes.com/2008/08/26/health/research/26rick.html

Ramsey-Goldman, Rosalind, Julie E. Dunn, Cheng-Fang Huang, Dorothy Dunlop, Joan E. Rairie, Shirley Fitzgerald, and Susan Manzi. 1999. Frequency of fractures in women with systemic lupus erythematosus: Comparison with United States population data. *Arthritis & Rheumatism* 42(5): 882-890.

Risk factors for pancreatic cancer. Accessed September 28, 2008 from http://www.oncologychannel.com/pancreaticcancer/index.shtml.

Risk of death increases after hip fracture. HealthinAging website. Accessed October 17, 2008 from http://www.healthinaging.org/aginginthek-now/research_content.asp?id=88.

Robsahm, Trude Eid, Steinar Tretli, Arne Dahlback, et al. 2004. Vitamin D3 from sunlight may improve the prognosis of breast-, colon- and prostate cancer (Norway). *Cancer Causes and Control* 15: 149-158.

Robsahm, Trude, S. Tretli, A. Dahlback. 2004. Vitamin D3 from sunlight may improve the prognosis of breast, colon and prostate cancer (Nor-way). *Cancer Causes and Control* 15: 149-158.

Robien, Kim, Gretchen J. Cutler, and DeAnn Lazovich. 2007. Vitamin D intake and breast cancer risk in postmenopausal women: The Iowa wom-en's health study. *Cancer Causes Control* 18: 775-782.

Rostand, Stephen G. 1997. 1997. Ultraviolet light may contribute to geographic and racial blood pressure differences. *Hypertension* 30: 150-156.

Sachan, Alok , Renu Gupta, Vinita Das, Anjoo Agarwal, Pradeep K Awasthi, and Vijayalakshmi Bhatia. 2005 (May). High prevalence of vitamin D deficiency among pregnant women and their newborns in northern India. *American Journal of Clinical Nutrition* 81(5): 1060-1064.

Salazar-Martinez Eduardo, Eduardo Lazcano-Ponce, Guillermo Gonzalez Lira-Lira, Escudero-Pedro Escudero-De los Rios, and Mauricio Hernandez-Avila. 2002. Nutritional determinants of epithelial ovarian cancer risk: a case-control study in Mexico. *Oncology* 63: 151-157.

Sardi, Bill. 2006. Is fibromyalgia just a vitamin D deficiency?

Trivedi, Daksha P., Richard Doll, and Kay Tee Khaw. 2003 (march). Effect of four monthly oral vitamin D3 (cholecalciferol) supplementation on fractures and mortality in men and women living in the community. *British Medical Journal* 326: 469-472.

Scragg, Robert, MaryFran Sowers, Colin Bell. December 2004, Serum 25-hydroxyvitamin D, diabetes and ethnicity in the third National Health and Nutrition Examination Survey. *Diabetes Care*, Vol. 27, Number 12,

Semba, Richard D., Elizabeth Garrett, Brent A. Johnson, Jack M. Guralnik, and Linda P. Fried. 2000. Vitamin D deficiency among older women with and without disability. *American Journal of Clinical Nutrition.* 72: 1529-1534.

Seventh Report by the Joint National Committee on Prevention, Detection, Evaluation and Treatment of High Blood Pressure. NIH Publication 03-5233, December 2003. Accessed January 4, 2009 from http://www.nhlbi.nih.gov/guidelines/hypertension/express.pdf.

Side Effects of Bisphosphonates. Epocrates Drug Database, (www.epocrates.com).

Skinner, Halcyon, G., Dominique, S. Michaud, Edward Giovannucci, et al. 2006 (September). Vitamin D Intake and the risk for pancreatic cancer in two cohort studies. *Cancer Epidemiology Biomarkers Prevention* 15(9): 1688-1695.

Smith Ellen. L., S. H. Pincus, L. Donovan, M. F. Holick. 1988 (September). A novel approach for the evaluation and treatment of psoriasis. Oral or topical use of 1,25-dihydroxyvitamin D3 can be a safe and effective therapy for psoriasis. *Journal of the American Academy of Dermatology* 19(3): 516-28.

Swezey, R L., and J. Adams. 1999 (December). Fibromyalgia: A risk factor for osteoporosis. *Journal of Rheumatology* 26(12): 2642-4.

Stene, L.C, J. Ulriksen, P. Magnus and G. Joner, Use of cod liver oil during pregnancy associated with lower risk of Type I diabetes in the offspring. (2000) *Diabetologia,* Vol 43, 1093:1098.

Teng Ming, Myles Wolf, M. Norma Ofsthun, et al. 2005. Activated injectable vitamin D and hemodialyisis survival: A historical cohort study. *Journal of the American Society of Nephrology* 16: 1115-1125.

Tseng, Marilyn, Rosalind A. Breslow, Barry I Graubard, and Regina G. Ziegler. 2005. Dairy, calcium and vitamin d intakes and prostate cancer risk in the national health and nutrition examination epidemiologic follow up study cohort. *American Journal of Clinical Nutrition* 2005; 81: 1147-1154.

Tuohimaa, Pentii, Leena Tenkannen, Heimo Syvala, et al. 2007 (February). Interactions of factors related to metabolic syndrome and vitamin D on risk of prostate cancer. *Cancer Epidemiology Biomarkers Prevention* 16(2): 1147-1154.

Tworoger, Shelley D., I-Min Lee, Julie E. Buring, et al. 2007 (April). Plasma 25-hydroxvitamin hydroxvitamin D and 1,25,- dihydroxvitamin dihydroxvitamin D and risk of incident ovarian cancer. *Cancer Epidemiology Biomarkers Prevention* 16(4): 783-788.

Uitterlinder, Andre, Stuart H. Ralston, Maria Luisa Brandi, et al. 2006. The association between common vitamin D receptor gene variations and osteoporosis: A participant level meta analysis. *Annals of Internal Medicine* 145: 255-264.

United States Renal Data System. *USRDS 2007 Annual Data Report*. Bethesda, MD: National Institute of Diabetes and Digestive and Kidney Diseases, National Institutes of Health, U.S. Department of Health and Human Services; 2007.

U.S. Renal Data System, USRDS 2008 Annual Data Report: Atlas of Chronic Kidney Disease and End-Stage Renal Disease in the United States, National Institutes of Health, National Institute of Diabetes and Digestive and Kidney Diseases, Bethesda, MD, 2008.

Vainio H., F. Bianchini. 2000. Cancer-preventive effects of sunscreens are uncertain. *Scand J Work Environ Health* 26(6): 529-531.

VanAmerongen, B M, C. D. Dijkstra, P. Lips, and C. H. Polman, 2004. Multiple sclerosis and vitamin D: An update. *European Journal of Clinical Nutrition* 58, 1095–1109.

Vieth, Reinhold. 1999. Vitamin D supplementation, 25-hydroxyvitamin D concentrations and safety. *American Journal of Clinical Nutrition* 69: 842-856.

Vieth Reinhold. 2006. What is the optimal vitamin D level for health? *Progress in Biophysics and Molecular Biology*, 92(1): 26-32.

Vitamin D status during pregnancy affects baby's dental health. 2008 (July). *Doctors Guide* Accessed November 29th, 2008 from http://www.docguide.com/news/content.nsf/news/852571020057CCF68525747B00689803.

Wactawski-Wende, Jean, AR. Assaf, KL Margolis.Calcium plus Vitamin D Supplementation and the Risk of Colorectal Cancer. The New England Journal of Medicine 354:7, February 16th 2006 pages 684-697

Walsh, Nancy. 2004 (November). Vitamin D Deficiency Found Common in RA Patients. *Family Practice News* 34(22):53.

Wang, Thomas J., Michael J. Pencina, Sarah L. Booth, Paul F. Jacques, et al. 2008. Vitamin D deficiency and risk of cardiovascular disease. *Circulation* 117: 503-511.

Washington Post. 2008 (June). Accessed September, 24, 2008 from http://www.washingtonpost.com/wp-dyn/content/article/2008/06/03/AR2008060301125.html

Watson, J. D., and F. H. C. Crick. 1953 (April). Molecular structures of nucleic acids: A structure for deoxyribose nucleic acid, *Nature* 171: 757-758. Accessed on November 28, 2008 from http://www.nature.com/nature/dna50/watsoncrick.pdf.

Weisberg, P. K.S. Scanlon, R. Li, and M. E. Cogswell. 2004. Nutritional rickets among children in the United States: Review of cases reported between 1986 and 2003. *American Journal of Clinical Nutrition.* 80: 1697S-1705S.

Westerdahl J; C. Ingvar A. Masback, H. Olsson. (2000). Sunscreen use and malignant melanoma. *International Journal of Cancer* 87: 145–50.

White, Linda. 2008 (February/March). Vitamin D: sunshine and so much more. *Mother Earth News.* Accessed on January 12, 2009 from http://www.motherearthnews.com/Natural-Health/2008-02-01/Vitamin-D-Sunshine-Supplements.aspx.

World Health Organization. Global cancer rates could increase by 50% to 15 million by 2020. Worldwide Cancer deaths 7 million. Accessed October 25th 2008 from http://www.who.int/mediacentre/news/releases/2003/pr27/en/.

Wortsman, Jacobo, Lois T. Matsuoka, Tai C. Chen, Zhiren Li, and Michael Holick. 2000. Decreased bioavailability of vitamin D in obesity. *American Journal of Clinical Nutrition* 72: 690-693.

Wyshak, Grace. 2000 (June). Teenaged girls, carbonated beverage consumption, and bone fractures. *Arch Pediatr Adolesc Med* 154:610-613._

Zhou, Wei, Rebecca Suk, Geoffrey Liu, et al. 2005 (October). Vitamin D is associated with improved survival in early-stage non small cell lung cancer. *Cancer Epidemiology Biomarkers Prev* 14(10): .

Zimmet, P., K. G. Alberti, and J. Shaw. 2001. Global and societal implications of the diabetes epidemic. *Nature* 414: 782-787.

Zoler, Mithcell. (1 July 2006), Low Vitamin D May Elevate Hypertension Risk. Family Practice News Vol. 36, Issue 13.

APPENDIX A

Recommended online retailers to purchase vitamin D3:

Drugstore.com

eHealthSupplies.com 1-800-471-7347

General Nutrition Centers (www.GNC.com)

Life Extension Foundation (www.lef.org) 1-800-544-4440

VitaCost (www.vitacost.com) 1-800-381-0759

Vitamin Shoppe (www.vitaminshoppe.com) 866-293-3367

APPENDIX B

Disease Incidence Prevention by Serum 25(OH)D Level

Chart prepared by Garland CF, Baggerly CA

Legend:
All percentages reference a common baseline of 25 ng/ml as shown on the chart.
%'s reflect the disease prevention % at the beginning and ending of available data. Example: Breast cancer incidence is reduced by 30% when the serum level is 34 ng/ml vs the baseline of 25 ng/ml. There is an 83% reduction in incidence when the serum level is 50 ng/ml vs the baseline of 25 ng/ml.
The x's in the bars indicate reasonable extrapolations from the data but are beyond existing data.

References:
All Cancers: Lappe JM, et al. Am J Clin Nutr. 2007;85:1586-91. Breast: Garland CF, Gorham ED, Mohr SB, Grant WB, Garland FC. Breast cancer risk according to serum 25-Hydroxyvitamin D. Meta-analysis of Dose-Response (abstract) American Association for Cancer Research Annual Meeting, 2008. Reference serum 25(OH)D was 5 ng/ml. Garland CF, et al. Amer Assoc Cancer Research Annual Mtg, April 2008. Colon: Gorham ED, et al. Am J Prev Med. 2007;32:210-6. Diabetes: Hypponen E, et al. Lancet 2001;358:1500-3. Endometrium: Mohr SB, et al. Prev. Med. 2007;45:323-4. Falls: Broe KE, et al. J Am Geriatr Soc. 2007;55:234-9. Fractures: Bischoff-Ferrari HA, et al. JAMA. 2005;293:2257-64. Heart Attack: Giovannucci et al. Arch Intern Med Vol 168 (No 11) June 9, 2008. Multiple Sclerosis: Munger KL, et al. JAMA. 2006;296:2832-8. Non-Hodgkin's Lymphoma: Purdue MP, et al. Cancer Causes Control. 2007;18:989-99. Ovary: Tworoger SS, et al. Cancer Epidemiol Biomarkers Prev. 2007;16:783-8. Renal: Mohr SB, et al. Int J Cancer. 2006;119:2705-9. Rickets: Arnaud SB.
Copyright GrassrootsHealth 10/16/08 www.grassrootshealth.org

Vitamin D Disease Incidence Chart use with permission from Carole Baggerly, Grassrootshealth.org. Chart compiled by Carole Baggerly and Dr. Cedric Garland.

205

INDEX

C

H

M

Madrid MD, Eric · iv, 8, 28, 40, 46, 68, 142, 168
magnesium · 57, 76, 92, 94
Mahoney, Diana · 112
mammogram · 118, 128
Martinez, Maria Elena · 138, 190
McAlindon, Timothy · 80
medical students · 8, 9, 169
Medicare · 73, 74
Melamed, Michael L. · 53, 97, 190, 191, 192
melanocytes · 157, 158, 161
Melanoma · 23, 119, 157, 161, 171, 191
Melanus, Persian Physician · 18
Mellanby, Edward · 17
Merck · 2, 17, 21, 69, 80, 81, 151, 152, 191
Merewood, Anne · 37, 191
methotrexate · 115
milnacipran
 Savella · 81
Moan, Johan · 159, 192
Mohr, Sharif B. · 123, 180
Moores Cancer Center · 131, 134, 159
Morimoto, S. · 115, 192
mortality, related to vitamin D · 34
Mudpies in Haiti ·
multiple sclerosis
 MS · 55, 110, 184, 193, 194
Munger, Kassandra L. · 110, 193

N

National Multiple Sclerosis Society · 109
National Osteoporosis Foundation · 58, 60, 63, 71, 193
New England Journal of Medicine · 51, 71, 78, 141, 177, 186, 187, 201
 NEJM · 60
Ng, Kimmie · 143
Nicolaysen, Ragnar · 26
Nieves, Jeri · 110, 194
Nobel Prize · ix, 17
Non-Hodgkin's lymphoma
 NHL · 119, 120, 163
Nonn, Larisa · 147, 187, 194

O

P

T

U

V